D1015259

Trail Map to Wellness Series

Leave Cancer in the Dust

Kristina Sampson

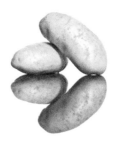

Cover design and interior page layout by William Sampson, Studio 5 Degrees.
Edited by Barbara McNichol, Barbara McNichol Editorial.

Leave Cancer in the Dust: 50 Tips to Prevent Breast Cancer and Supercharge Your Health.

Kristina Sampson – First Edition: May 2014
Printed in the United States of America
ISBN: 978-0985072780
Library of Congress Control Number: 2014937746

Visit www.thevaildiet.com

The author and publisher endeavor to make the information in this book accurate and up to date. It is a general guide. Before taking action on medical, legal, or financial matters, you should consult with qualified professionals who can help you consider your unique circumstances. The author and publisher cannot accordingly accept any liability for any loss or damage suffered as a consequence of relying on the information contained in this book.

Mention of specific leaders in research, education, therapy, or other authorities in this book does not imply they endorse this book. Internet addresses are accurate at the time of printing.

Dedication

For my husband,

JOHN,

who will happily eat anything I serve him and say it's delicious.
Thank you for giving me a safe space to pursue my dreams.

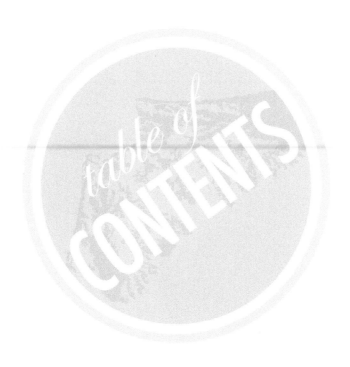

table of CONTENTS

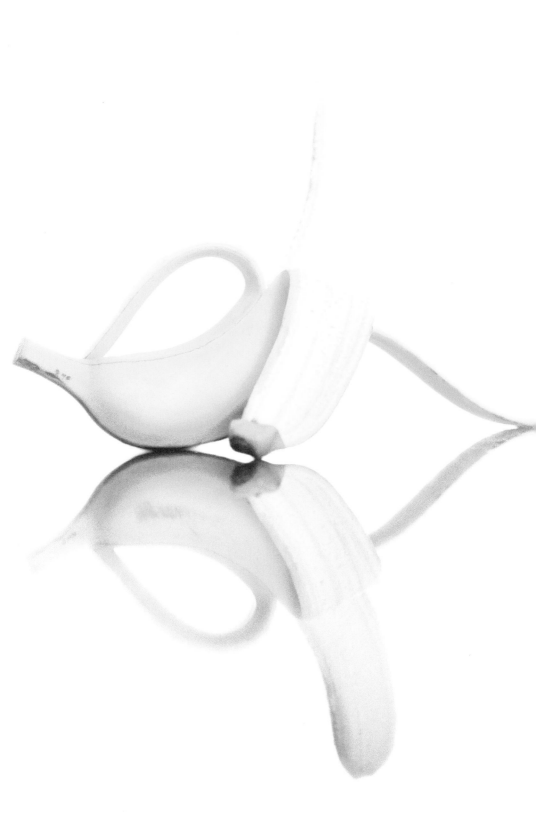

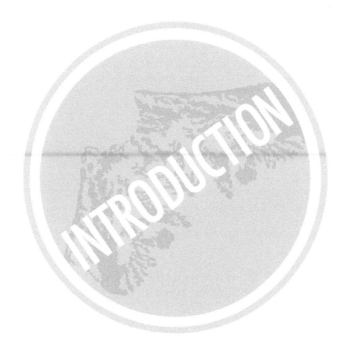

Welcome, fellow wellness enthusiast. I am thrilled you have taken this *big* step in embracing your health. The tips you'll learn in this book — *if you apply them* — will help you take proactive steps to not only prevent breast cancer but supercharge your health overall.

With the exception of skin cancer, breast cancer is the most common cancer in American women. Over 232,000 new cases of invasive breast cancer were diagnosed among women in the U.S. in 2013, along with an additional 64,000+ cases of ductal carcinoma in situ (commonly referred to as "DCIS"). More than 2,000 cases of breast cancer in men were diagnosed. Sadly, about 40,000 people died from this disease in 2013.[1]

Since my own breast cancer diagnosis in 2007, I have researched how to prevent this disease — some things I was already doing and others I wish I had known years ago. What steps can you take to protect yourself from being among these statistics?

This book includes 50 of the most promising breast cancer prevention tips discovered to date. Some of these tried-and-true tips are supported by years of research; others are new and exciting discoveries.

In this book you'll read about:

- 🌸 25 foods that nourish your body and significantly lower your risk of breast cancer,

- 🌸 15 ways to reduce your exposure to dangerous foods, chemicals, and environmental factors that increase your risk of breast cancer and damage your health in other ways,

- 🌸 5 tips to "shake your booty" and help your body reap the rewards of physical activity, and

- 🌸 5 practices to quiet your mind, reduce stress, and find your bliss.

Add to these *5 bonus detoxification tips* to give your body a boost in getting rid of the toxins it's exposed to every day.

Most important, get ready to discover ways to safely and easily incorporate these 50+ ideas into your life.

You'll find a wealth of information in this book. It may be overwhelming to incorporate all of these tips into your life at once. Instead, select one each week and make a whole-hearted effort to build it into your life *for that week.*

That's it. If you don't enjoy this one new practice or it doesn't resonate with you, move on to one that does. Voilà! With 50 tips instead of 52, you even get a two-week break for the holidays!

Suggestion: Throughout the year, sprinkle in the bonus detox tips when you feel you haven't been as kind to your body as usual, or when it might need extra help.

My Story

"You have breast cancer." *Pow!*

"It's grade three." *Wham!*

"It's triple negative." *Whack!*

"I'm sorry, but it has spread to your lymph nodes." *Ka-boom!*

Those were the words I heard beginning on July 3, 2007, and over the days and weeks that followed.

Yes, fireworks went off that year—but not the celebratory kind.

But unlike most people, I didn't think, "Why me?" What popped into my mind instead was, "Of course I have cancer."

You see, cancer and I go way back. At the young age of 25, I was diagnosed with a malignant tumor on my spinal cord. So the delusion that cancer wouldn't ever happen to me had been wiped out early. I went through a risky surgery followed by 30 radiation treatments and five years of holding my breath. Would the cancer return?

Eventually, though, I (sort of) forgot about it, moved to New York City, and went about my life. But I never *quite* forgot.

Ten years later, in 2005, I moved from New York to Vail, Colorado. Shortly after, I located a nearby cancer center and had a nagging suspicion I'd become intimately familiar with it one day.

Unfortunately, my premonition came true—but this time, I knew more.

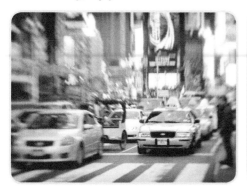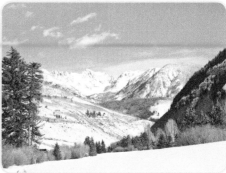

Nutrition has always been an important part of my life.
My parents were "health food nuts" since the 1970s. Eating healthy foods has gone from a *mild interest* in my 20s to a *strong awareness* when my first cancer was diagnosed to a raging passion today.

What I have learned has helped me immensely. And it can help you transform your life, whether you have cancer or not.

Specifically, I've learned that food is a medicine that can change our bodies, even our genes. Yes, we have an army of cancer fighters at our disposal: broccoli, kale, blueberries, and all their medicinal buddies. Armed with vitamins, minerals, and phytonutrients, these warriors are ready to fight off cancer before this disease ever gets a chance to take hold.

No need to wait. Given my own breast cancer diagnosis, I continue to fight against the cancer-producing elements in my life. And I've never felt better.

Are you ready to fight, too?

My Philosophy

The days following my breast cancer diagnosis remain fresh in my mind. Perhaps it could be called denial, but I didn't focus on what was going to happen *to* me. Instead, my thoughts revolved around what I was going to *make* happen.

My mantra became "I'll come out the other side of this healthier and happier than before, and with better relationships with those around me."

Yes, I knew I was in for a long, bumpy ride. But I took over the driver's seat without a moment's hesitation.

Now, my health-food-nut parents weren't (and still aren't) big fans of traditional medicine. In our household, we always looked for a natural remedy first. As a result, I'm a big believer in holistic and alternative medicine. However, I also have a healthy respect for science and believe that traditional medicine has its place. In my own cancer treatments, I have received a combination of traditional and alternative therapies that have all served me well.

Still, I'm bothered by the fact that scientific studies aren't foolproof. They can be, and often are, manipulated.

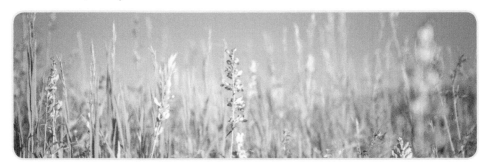

Have you ever noticed how often studies funded by corporations or industries support whichever outcome lines their pocketbook? And frankly, traditional Western medicine has been on the wrong side of history too many times to assume it always knows what's right.

Remember, only a couple of generations ago doctors would walk into a treatment room *holding a cigarette* and saying smoking wasn't dangerous. Today, far too many doctors believe there is no connection between the food we eat and our health. But as happened with cigarette smoking, history will prove them wrong.

Experts say that only 5 to 10 percent of cancers are based in genetics; the remaining 90 to 95 percent relate to environment and lifestyle. Of those, 25 to 30 percent are linked to tobacco use, 30 to 35 percent to diet, and 10 to 15 percent to infection. The remaining cases stem from stress, lack of physical activity, and exposure to toxins in the environment.[2]

Addressing the 30 to 35 percent related to diet, I say society's 50-year experiment with overeating fast, cheap, and convenient processed "food" has failed miserably. Our population gets fatter and sicker by the minute.

It's time to start supercharging our health-both as individuals and as a society!

How? It starts at a grassroots level one person at a time. Each of us can drive the factors that affect our own health. We can influence the big corporations that get us addicted to bad foods as well as the hospitals and pharmaceutical companies that profit from keeping us sick. And we can certainly apply the tips throughout this book as much as possible.

Please join me in the driver's seat. Let's get started.

A Word About Organics

Let's talk organic vs. conventional. If you have an interest in food, you probably heard about the 2012 study conducted by Stanford University.[3] It concluded that organic vegetables and fruits were no more nutritious than their conventional counterparts. To put it mildly, this study raised "holy H-E-double hockey sticks."

Since its release, the study has been criticized by many in the health field. One reason involves researchers not looking at all nutrients but only certain ones in which the difference between organic and conventional tends to be small. They ignored others in which much larger variations have been shown.

In addition, even though the researchers found low pesticide levels on the organic produce, they glossed over that fact when reporting their results.

A similar study came to the exact opposite conclusion—that is, organic vegetables and fruits do, in fact, contain more nutrients than their conventional counterparts.[4]

Despite what any study says, I don't want pesticides in my body. Pesticides are designed to kill; that's all I need to know. Plus, they pose far more danger to the tiny bodies of children than grown-ups.

To minimize pesticide exposure for you and your family, use the checklist on the following page from the Environmental Working Group's 2014 Shopper's Guide to Pesticides in Produce (www.ewg.org/foodnews) to help you make wise choices. Take extra time to peel or thoroughly wash conventional produce from the "Dirty Dozen"—fruits and vegetables that have the most pesticides. Most important, though, is to eat lots of fruits and vegetables, organic or not.

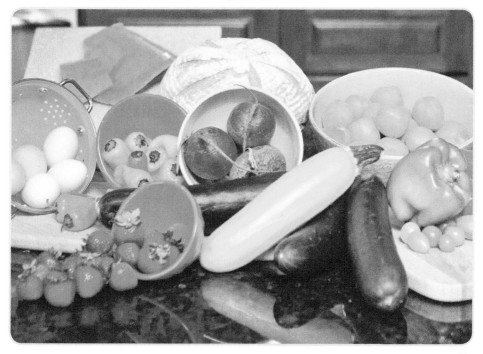

Dirty Dozen Plus™

1 Apples

2 Strawberries

3 Grapes

4 Celery

5 Peaches

6 Spinach

7 Sweet Bell Peppers

8 Nectarines (imported)

9 Cucumbers

10 Cherry Tomatoes

11 Snap Peas (imported)

12 Potatoes

13 Hot Peppers

14 Kale/Collard Greens

Note: These are the fruits and veggies with the most pesticide residue. Try to buy organic or at the very least, peel or wash thoroughly.

Clean Fifteen™

1 Avocados

2 Sweet Corn

3 Pineapples

4 Cabbage

5 Sweet peas (frozen)

6 Onions

7 Asparagus

8 Mangos

9 Papayas

10 Kiwi

11 Eggplant

12 Grapefruit

13 Cantaloupe

14 Cauliflower

15 Sweet potatoes

Note: These are the fruits and veggies with the least pesticide residue. Organic is great if you can afford it, but don't sweat it - conventional is fine for most of these. Take caution with sweet corn and papaya as these are often genetically modified; organic is your safest bet.

Discovery Center

Do-It-Yourself Fruit and Veggie Wash

Like germs and bacteria, pesticide residue can't be removed by water alone. Instead, mix and use this low-cost spray that works well:

- ❀ 8 ounces water
- ❀ ½ cup white vinegar (the cheap stuff will do)
- ❀ ⅓ cup natural, chemical-free soap or dish soap (Dr. Bronner's and Mrs. Meyers brands are great options)

Pour all ingredients into a 16-ounce spray bottle and shake. Spray on fruits and veggies, rub vigorously, and rinse with water. Wiping your fruits and veggies with a paper towel after washing will remove even more pesticide residue.

Note: Be sure to thoroughly wash produce even when you will not eat the skin. During slicing, the blade of your knife can carry nasty germs from the outside of the skin to the edible flesh.

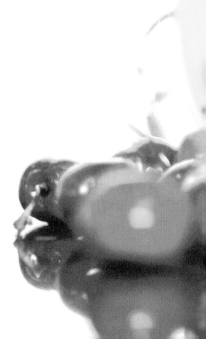

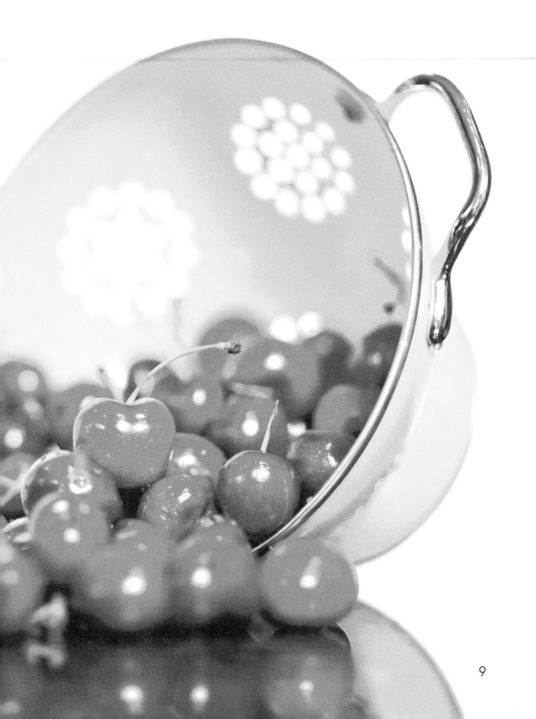

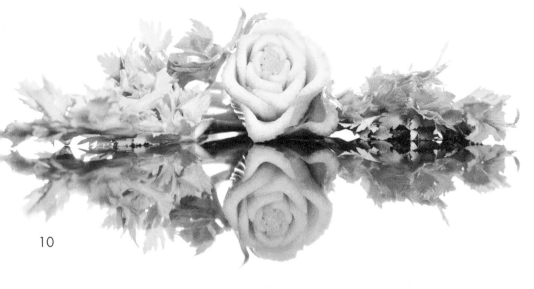

10

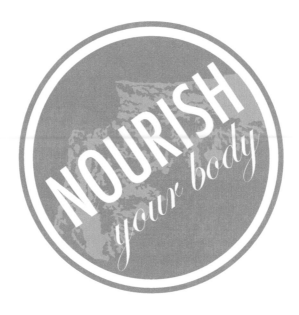

As noted, 30 to 35 percent of cancer cases are believed to be caused by eating an unhealthy diet. That means of the more than 1,000,000 cases of cancer diagnosed in the U.S. each year, over 300,000 of them are likely preventable through changes in diet alone. That also means more than 300,000 people a year don't have to go through surgery, chemotherapy, or radiation—or even die from the disease. Yes, *every* year.

Can any single food by itself protect you against cancer? That's unknown. However, regularly eating a combination of nourishing foods—and avoiding others—can offer significant protection against the disease.

Study after study has shown the best diet for cancer prevention is primarily based on eating plant foods, including a wide variety of vegetables, fruits, beans, whole grains, nuts, and seeds. Because excessive protein intake has been linked to cancer, animal proteins such as meat, poultry, or dairy are best eaten in moderation.

Among the veggies and fruits you can choose from, which are the best ones for reducing your risk of getting breast cancer? Which should you avoid? Read on!

Veggies

Can't Beat Beets

Beets belong to the same family as chard, spinach, and quinoa; they're native to the Mediterranean region. Used medicinally and as dyes for centuries before becoming popular as a food in the 19th century, beets were brought to America by the colonists. In the U.S., the most common types consumed are the red, yellow, and gold varieties. (Much of our table sugar comes from a different variety of beet known as the sugar beet.)

Beets contain an antioxidant called betalain. This not only gives them their beautiful red color but, according to research, may starve tumors and inhibit the division of cancer cells. In animal studies, beet extract has been shown to reduce cancers of the esophagus, lung, skin, and colon.[5] In laboratory studies on human tumor cells, one particular betalain called betanin has been linked to reductions in cancers of the breast, colon, stomach, lung, and central nervous system.[6]

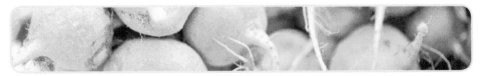

The health benefits of beets don't stop there. Beets are anti-inflammatory and provide a good source of folate, magnesium, potassium, iron, fiber, carotenoids, and melatonin. (Melatonin is associated with a lower risk of breast cancer.) Beets also increase blood flow, decrease blood pressure, protect the liver, and aid your body's natural detoxification processes.

You want to cook beets by roasting or steaming them. However, as with many veggies, the beneficial compounds in beets are heat sensitive. So you can minimize betalain damage and retain the "good stuff" by steaming beets for 15 minutes or less, or roasting them for one hour or less. Juice raw beets to gain their healthy goodness without the worries of any heat damage.

Discovery Center
Don't Ditch the Greens

To get the most nutritional bang for your buck, don't forget the greens growing out of the top of your beets.

Beet greens provide a great source of lutein, a powerful antioxidant and anti-inflammatory compound shown to decrease the risk of certain types of cancer.

Beet greens can be lightly sautéed or juiced.

---

② Choose Celery

Celery originated in the Mediterranean region and has been grown for medicinal purposes for thousands of years. It's a member of the *Apiaceae* family (along with carrots, coriander, cilantro, cumin, dill, fennel, parsnip, parsley, and about 3,700 other species of plants). European colonists brought celery to America, but it's not known exactly when. Today, most of this veggie grown in the U.S. comes from California.

Celery contains a compound called apigenin. Researchers have discovered that this substance can shrink a type of tumor caused by a particularly deadly, fast-growing human breast cancer cell. The compound induces apoptosis (programmed cell death, a naturally occurring process in the body), inhibits cell growth, and reduces the expression of the HER2/neu gene associated with a more aggressive type of breast cancer. These results were achieved with no toxic side effects.[7]

Apigenin is so promising that clinical trials could start immediately. However, as one of the researchers involved in this study stated, "Since apigenin is easily extracted from plants, pharmaceutical companies don't stand to profit from the treatment; hence the industry won't put money into studying something you can grow in your garden."[8]

Apigenin is also found in several other herbs such as basil, cilantro, oregano, parsley, and tarragon as well as certain fruits, vegetables, tea, and beans. In addition to apigenin, celery provides vitamin K and contains several vitamins and minerals. It also has almost no calories and may reduce one's LDL (bad) cholesterol and blood pressure. An alkalizing substance, it's also an anti-inflammatory and aids in digestion.

I suggest including plenty of celery in your diet. This versatile veggie can be added to casseroles, soups, stews, or other cooked dishes. You can also eat it raw in salads or as a snack on its own.

Make celery a "must" in your fresh green juices because a green juice without celery is like a day without sunshine!

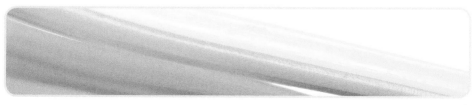

Ants on a Log

This perennial favorite of Girl Scout troops all over makes a pleasing, nutritious, protein-packed snack. And it's a great way to add celery to your diet.

- ❀ Celery stalks
- ❀ Nut butter of your choice (almond butter is fantastic!)
- ❀ Raisins (or other dried fruit of your choice)

Spread nut butter in the hollow section of the celery stalk and top with dried fruit. For variety, you could substitute hummus and seasoned pumpkin seeds. Enjoy!

Crave Cruciferous Vegetables

Cruciferous vegetables are widely cultivated all over the world. These veggies include arugula, bok choy, broccoli, Brussels sprouts, cabbage, cauliflower, collard greens, horseradish, kale, mustard greens, radish, turnip, watercress, and several others. Their name comes from their four-petal flower that resembles a cross or "crucifer."

Cruciferous veggies are loaded with phytonutrients as well as important vitamins, minerals, and fiber. One of these nutrients, sulforaphane, is a compound shown to protect against cell damage as well as selectively target and kill cancer cells. In one study, sulforaphane was also shown to reduce the number of breast cancer stem cells in mice—a crucial effect because chemotherapy does *not* work against breast cancer stem cells.[9]

Another recent study showed that women who ate the most cruciferous vegetables had significantly lower rates of breast cancer recurrence (35 percent) or death from the disease (62 percent) than those who ate the least.[10]

In addition to cancer-fighting sulforaphane, cruciferous vegetables are loaded with vitamins A, C, K, folate, and fiber. These superstars are also rich in minerals such as magnesium, manganese, phosphorus, potassium, selenium, and zinc.

Believe it or not, cruciferous vegetables are also a good source of protein, with broccoli actually containing more protein per calorie than steak.

However, sulforaphane is killed by excessive heat. So cook or steam cruciferous vegetables lightly for only three to four minutes, allowing most of the nutrients to remain intact. Don't boil your veggies, cruciferous or otherwise (except maybe potatoes); they lose far too many nutrients this way. Opinions vary on whether or not microwaving is safe for you or your food. Some experts believe a significant amount of nutrients are lost and others state that microwaving vegetables retains far more nutrients than boiling. At the very least, do not microwave in plastic as this may potentially release endocrine disruptors.

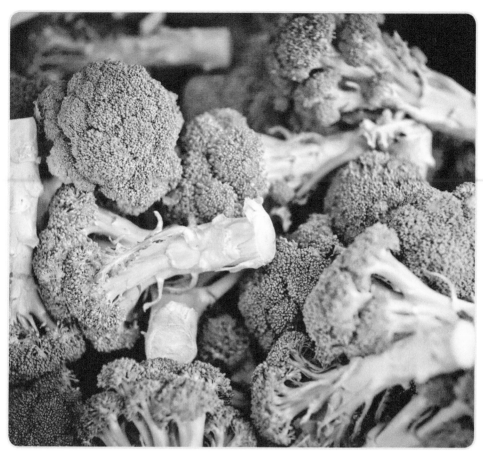

At a minimum, include a variety of cruciferous veggies in your diet two or three times a week. Better yet, aim for five or more times. And to increase the amount of sulforaphane to out-of-this-world levels, enjoy broccoli sprouts. They're easy to eat raw and contain 10 to 100 times the amount of sulforaphane as mature broccoli.

Live by this motto: "Never, ever, pass up broccoli."

Discovery Center

A Word About Watercress

Recent research has shown that the compound phenylethyl isothiocyanate in watercress, a cruciferous veggie, may suppress the development of breast cancer cells by starving them of their blood and oxygen supplies.[11] Watercress is also good source of folate, vitamins A, C, E, and K, and minerals such as calcium, copper, manganese, magnesium, phosphorus, and potassium.

Enjoy eating watercress raw as a delicious addition to any salad or sandwich. It's also wonderful on pizza or in soups and other cooked dishes.

Cruciferous Veggies - Cooked or Raw?

Since the early 1980s, experts have been debating whether cruciferous vegetables are best eaten raw or cooked. After all, consuming them raw allows all of the nutrients and enzymes to remain intact.

However, some experts claim that eating raw cruciferous vegetables can lead to problems such as goiter or hypothyroidism. Substances in cruciferous veggies called goitrogens, which are inactivated by heat, can potentially cause these issues.

More current research has shown that eating raw cruciferous vegetables is likely dangerous only for those who already have an impaired thyroid or iodine deficiency.

To get maximum benefit with the smallest amount of risk, follow these guidelines when eating cruciferous vegetables:

- ✿ Get your thyroid and iodine levels checked to ensure your thyroid is functioning properly and you don't have a deficiency in iodine.

- ✿ Avoid eating massive amounts of raw cruciferous vegetables.

- ✿ Rotate your choice of cruciferous vegetables to get a variety of nutrients without overdosing on any particular one.

- ✿ Watch for symptoms of hypothyroidism, such as fatigue, unexplained weight gain, dry skin, thinning hair, increased sensitivity to cold, and changes in the look or feel of your neck.

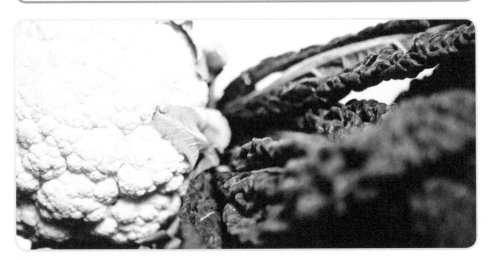

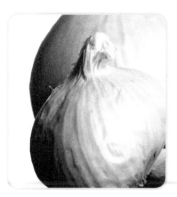
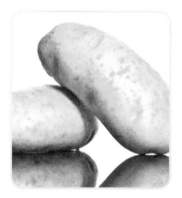
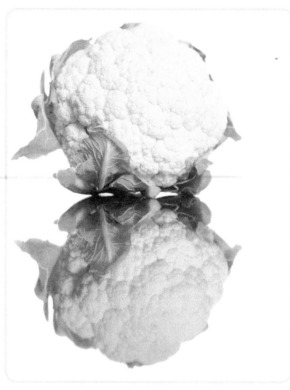

Garlic Mashed Potatoes and Cauliflower

This easy-peasy recipe is a great way to disguise cauliflower from your kids, or even your spouse! It also significantly cuts the calories in a typical mashed potato recipe. Serves 6-8.

- ❀ 1 head cauliflower, chopped into approximately 1-1½ inch pieces

- ❀ 2 large russet potatoes, peeled and cubed into 1-inch pieces

- ❀ 1 head roasted garlic, skins removed

- ❀ ¼ cup unsweetened non-dairy milk such as soy or almond

- ❀ ¼ cup Earth Balance organic buttery spread

- ❀ salt and pepper to taste

Boil potatoes and cauliflower together until easily pierced with a fork. Drain, add roasted garlic and buttery spread, and mash. Add milk, salt and pepper. Mix thoroughly with a hand mixer or manually.

Gorge on Garlic and Onions

Garlic and onions have been cultivated for several thousand years. They're believed to be native to Central Asia. However, some evidence suggests onions may have been first grown in Iran and Pakistan.

Garlic and onions are part of the *Allium* family, which includes chives, leeks, shallots, and scallions. These vegetables are rich in organosulfur compounds, which are believed to give these special vegetables their cancer-fighting abilities. A substance called allicin—formed when garlic and onions are chopped, crushed, or chewed— forms the protective sulfur compounds. Allicin also gives garlic and onions their pungent smell.

One large European study found a link between the consumption of onions and garlic and a decreased risk in breast cancer as well as cancers of the mouth, esophagus, colon, larynx, ovaries, and prostate. In fact, the study noted a 50 to 80 percent reduction of all major cancers.[12] In addition, a French study found a statistically significant decrease in breast cancer risk among those who ate the most onions, garlic, and fiber.[13]

Garlic and onions come with many additional health benefits. Both vegetables contain vitamins B6 and C as well as important minerals such as manganese, phosphorus, and copper. They are anti-inflammatory and can thin the blood, lower cholesterol, and reduce the risk of heart disease. Garlic is also antibacterial, antiviral, and antifungal.

Garlic and onions aren't high in pesticide residue, so you don't necessarily have to buy organic. Strive to eat least two cloves of garlic and one-half of an onion every day.

Make garlic, onions, and other alliums the foundation of your anti-cancer diet.

Discovery Center

Peeling and Chopping Onions and Garlic

Because the beneficial compounds in onions are concentrated toward the outside of the onion, remove as little of the edible portion on the outside as possible.

In addition, to maximize the anti-cancer benefits of both garlic and onions, either eat them raw or let them sit for at least 10 minutes after cutting or chopping. That's because allicin won't form when the veggies are being heated. But it's relatively heat-stable so if allicin is allowed to form before heating, many of its benefits will remain even after cooking. However, don't overcook either garlic or onions. Rather, cook them long enough to make them palatable to you.

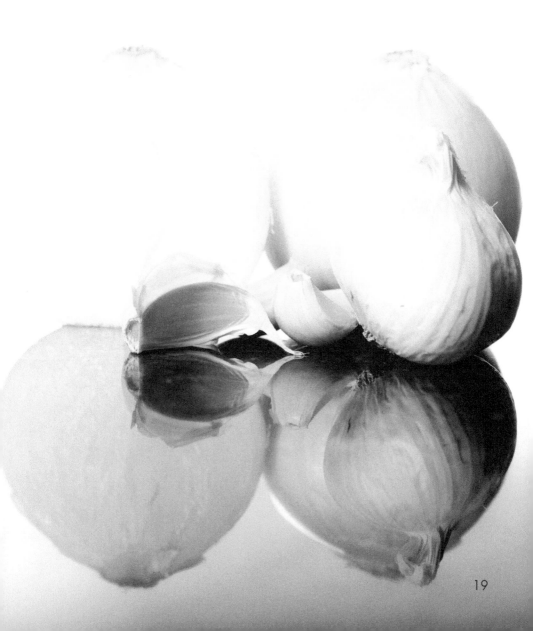

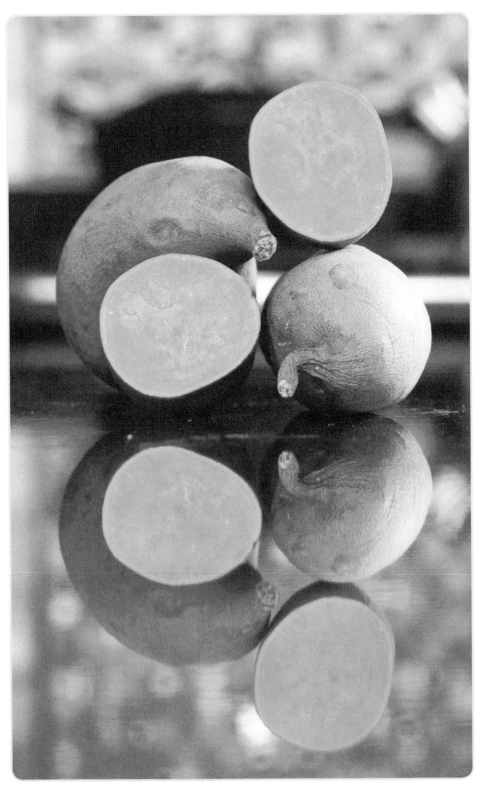

Seek Sweets (Sweet Potatoes, that is!)

Contrary to what the grocery store label says, those orange-fleshed, copper-skinned vegetables are not yams. They are sweet potatoes. (Yams aren't even related to sweet potatoes.)

Sweet potatoes come in hundreds of varieties and flesh colors, but the ones most common in the U.S. have either white or orange flesh. The USDA began labeling the orange ones as "yams" to avoid confusing the two (but I'm not sure that's working!). Sweet potatoes are believed to have originated in South America; today, North Carolina is the largest producer of the vegetable in the U.S.

Sweet potatoes are rich in carotenoids such as beta-carotene and other antioxidants that may fight breast cancer. One study found that women who eat a lot of vegetables containing beta-carotene, folate, vitamin C, and fiber—all of which are found in sweet potatoes—have about half the risk of breast cancer than those who don't eat these foods.[14]

Another study that analyzed the results of 18 other studies found that women who ate foods with carotenoids such as alpha-carotene, beta-carotene, and lutein had a lower risk of developing ER- breast cancer than women who didn't eat those foods.[15]

You can count on sweet potatoes as great sources of fiber, vitamins A, B, C, and E, folate, and minerals such as manganese, potassium, and copper. In fact, sweet potatoes contain more potassium than a banana.

This vegetable, an anti-inflammatory, contains a substance called chlorogenic acid that reduces insulin resistance. Studies have shown sweet potatoes may actually improve blood sugar in people with type-2 diabetes. In fact, this vegetable is such a nutritional superstar, the Center for Science in the Public Interest (CSPI) gave sweet potatoes the number one spot on its "10 Best Foods" list.[16]

When it comes to sweet potatoes, skip the white-fleshed variety and go for color. The darker the color, the more cancer-fighting beta-carotene the vegetable contains. Since sweet potatoes made the "Clean Fifteen" list, you don't necessarily have to buy organic.

I suggest eating the peel, which contains many nutrients and a lot of fiber that can slow down blood sugar reactions. If you plan to eat the peel, buying organic is optimal.

Discovery Center

How to Eat Your Sweets

Steam, boil, or bake your sweet potatoes. Just keep in mind that baked sweet potatoes have a higher glycemic index than boiled or steamed, possibly raising its blood sugar effects.

It's best to eat your sweet potato with a modest amount of fat to significantly increase your absorption of beta-carotene.

Fruits

 ## Adore Avocados

Surprising, yes. Avocado is a fruit! Stranger yet, it's actually a berry. Another interesting fact: avocado contains the most protein of any fruit, with about four grams per avocado.

Avocados originated in Central America and today, the vast majority of avocados grown in the U.S. come from California.

While avocado may not be a food you associate with cancer prevention, it contains a plethora of cancer-fighting phytonutrients including carotenoids, oleic acid, and glutathione peroxidase. (See Glossary on page 110.) According to Dr. Mark Hyman, glutathione is "the most important molecule you need to stay healthy and prevent aging, cancer, heart disease, dementia and more, and necessary to treat everything from autism to Alzheimer's disease."[17]

Another cancer-fighting nutrient in avocado is vitamin E. This important vitamin has been shown to slow or stop cancer cells from replicating as well as promote apoptosis. The Nurses Health study followed more than 80,000 women for over a decade. It showed that pre-menopausal women with a family history of breast cancer who ate the highest amounts of vitamin E had 43 percent fewer cases of the disease.[18] It's best to get your vitamin E from food rather than supplements.

As a bonus, avocados are not only great cancer fighters; they're also anti-inflammatory and rich in antioxidants, fiber, folate, and vitamins B6, C, and K. Plus, the fruit contains more potassium than a banana—important because less than 2 percent of American adults take in the recommended amount of potassium. Having enough potassium is crucial for regulating blood pressure levels every day.

There is no reason to be scared of the fat in avocados. Not only are avocados loaded with nutrients, their monounsaturated fats help your body absorb those nutrients. You're wise to eat a half or a whole small avocado every day.

Not sure how to add avocado to your diet? These tips can help you deliciously incorporate them into your daily eating:

- Go for guacamole. Delicious and easy to find, it's one of the healthiest items on many restaurant menus.

- Substitute mayonnaise with avocado on sandwiches and replace fats in baking with equal parts avocado. Bye-bye butter!

- ◆ Go crazy and use avocados in your desserts, making an amazing chocolate mousse and even ice cream.

Start at the beginner level, and you'll work your way up to being an avocado expert in no time.

Avocado Chocolate Mousse

Wow. That's all I can say about this yummy chocolate avocado mousse.

- ✿ 2 ripe avocados
- ✿ ⅓ cup organic cacao powder (no added sugar or artificial sweeteners)
- ✿ ¼ cup pure maple syrup
- ✿ ¼ cup almond milk
- ✿ 1 tbsp coconut oil
- ✿ 2 tsp vanilla extract or scrapings from one vanilla bean

Place all ingredients in a food processor and mix until smooth and creamy. Best enjoyed immediately. Avocados oxidize quickly, which will change the taste of this dessert...and not for the better!

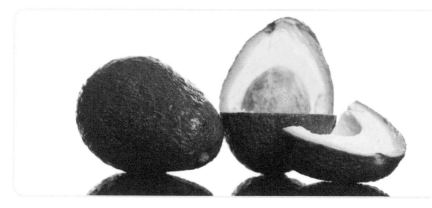

Avocados and Latex Allergies

The proteins that cause allergies to latex, which is derived from the sap of a rubber tree, are present in certain foods including avocado, banana, chestnut, kiwifruit, passionfruit, plum, strawberry, and tomato. Approximately 50 percent of those who have a latex allergy are also allergic to these foods.

If you have a latex allergy, take care before eating avocado or any of the other foods listed above.

Ask for Apples

Although apple pie is distinctively American, apples are not. Out of the thousands of different varieties of apples grown in the United States, only the crabapple is native. Europeans introduced additional species when they settled in America during the 17th century.

Apples are rich in phytochemicals—quercetin and others—that act as strong antioxidants. These compounds can prevent oxidative stress and inflammation in the body, both of which can damage genes and may cause cancer.

Apples are a good source of fiber and vitamin C. Laboratory studies have shown that the phytochemicals in apples can inhibit cancer cell growth. In addition, population studies have linked eating apples to a reduction in the risk of some cancers.[19]

In animal testing, one group of researchers fed rats apple extract equal to eating between one and six apples a day. The incidence of tumors in these rats fell between 25 and 61 percent lower than for rats *not* receiving apple extracts. In addition, a specific type of highly malignant tumor was found in 81 percent of the rats that didn't receive apple extracts, but only in 57 percent of rats receiving the equivalent of one apple per day, and 23 percent of rats receiving six apples. These same researchers found that apple extracts can boost the cancer-killing effects of chemotherapy drugs.[20]

Quick Eats

Cancer-Fighting Green Juice

This delicious green juice includes a plethora of cancer-fighting veggies, fruits, and spices. It's my go-to juice when I want a healthy pick-me-up.

- 1 cucumber (unpeeled if organic; peeled if conventional)
- 3 large celery stalks
- 1 small Granny Smith apple
- 1 broccoli stalk (lightly steamed and chilled if you have thyroid issues)
- ½ lemon, peeled
- ½ to 1-inch piece raw ginger

Use a juicer such as a Breville, Jack LaLanne, or Champion brand (there are tons of good juicers available at a wide range of price points).

This recipe can also be made as a green smoothie using a high-speed blender such as a Vitamix. Just peel the ginger, omit the broccoli stalk, and throw in a handful of your favorite leafy greens.

In addition to their potential cancer-fighting abilities, apples have been linked to the reduced risk of cardiovascular disease and diabetes in humans. This amazing fruit has also been shown to lower cholesterol, regulate blood sugar, and benefit our oh-so-important gut bacteria.

The old adage is true – an apple a day really DOES keep the doctor away!

Keep these important things in mind when eating apples:

- ❁ Processing can damage the phytochemicals in an apple, so it is best to eat the whole fruit rather than make juices, sauces, or pies. (Fresh juice is an exception, but stick to one apple to avoid getting too much sugar.)

- ❁ The peel of an apple contains two to three times the amount of flavonoids as the flesh, so it's best to eat fruit with its peel on. However, apples do occupy the #1 spot on the EWG's list of "The Dirty Dozen" for a reason. The peel may harbor considerable amounts of pesticide residue. If possible, buy organic. If not, wash your apples thoroughly or even peel them before eating.

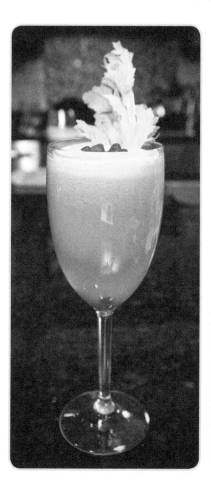
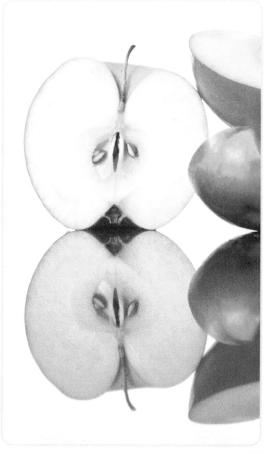

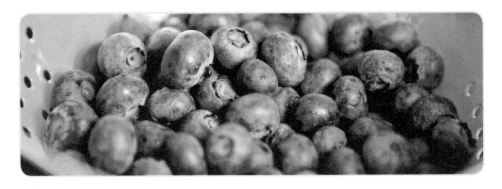

⑧ Binge on Blueberries

Unlike apples, blueberries are native to North America. They were an important part of the diet of Native Americans and early European settlers who even used them to make paint for their houses. Nowadays, blueberries are grown commercially in several dozen states; however, the vast majority of those available in the U.S. come from Maine.

Did you know that blueberries are among the most antioxidant-rich foods on the *planet*? They are also high in fiber and rich in vitamins and minerals including vitamin C, K, and manganese. On top of all that, they are a low-glycemic fruit that offers a lot in a mere 80 calories per cup.

Several studies have indicated amazing results for the effects of blueberries on breast cancer. One large study of almost 75,000 women showed that those who ate at least one serving a week of blueberries had a 31 percent lower risk of post-menopausal estrogen receptor negative (ER-) breast cancer than those who didn't.[21]

Note: While only 20 percent of breast cancers are ER-, they still make up a dispro-portionately large share of breast cancer deaths. Finally, good news for us ER- gals!

Another study found that blueberry juice held back the migration of triple-negative breast cancer cells. That means *it stopped the cancer from spreading*. The research-ers also found that blueberry extract shrank tumors, stopped cancer cells from multi-plying, and triggered apoptosis.[22]

Blueberries have also been shown to protect against other types of cancer including colon cancer. They can lower blood sugar, improve memory, protect the eyes from macular degeneration, blast belly fat, and reduce the risk of heart attack. Amazing!

At a minimum, eat one-half cup of blueberries several times a week. Enjoy them in smoothies, on cereal or oatmeal, baked into healthy muffins or breads, or simply plain.

When it comes to all types of berries, select organic. Residue from more than 50 types of pesticides has been detected on blueberries alone. However, to save money, you can buy your berries in bulk when they're in season during the summer and freeze for use all winter long. Costco and similar stores carry reasonably priced bags of frozen organic blueberries and other berries throughout the year.

Blueberry Superfood Smoothie

- ❀ 1½ cups unsweetened almond or other non-dairy milk

- ❀ 1 cup frozen blueberries (or 4-5 one-inch pieces of frozen banana and ½ cup frozen blueberries)

- ❀ 1 handful of fresh or frozen greens such as spinach or kale

- ❀ 1 scoop vegan vanilla protein powder

- ❀ 1 tablespoon chia or flax seed, or a combination of both

- ❀ ½ teaspoon cinnamon

- ❀ 1 tsp coconut oil or almond butter (optional)

- ❀ 1 tsp of maca, spirulina, or other powdered superfood (optional)

Blend for 1-2 minutes in a Vitamix or other powerful blender. Top with extra treats like cacao nibs, dried mulberries, or coconut flakes.

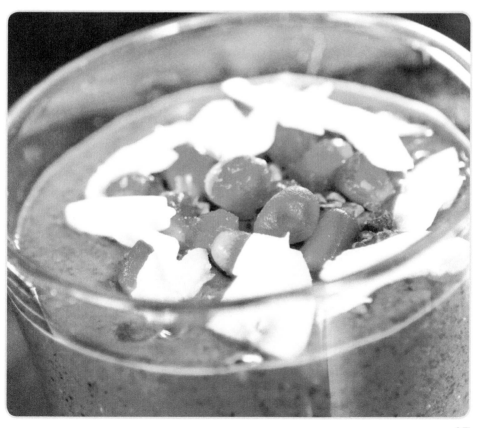

Pick Peaches and Nectarines

The stone fruits of peaches and nectarines are members of the rose family. In effect, nectarines are simply peaches without the fuzzy skin, a result of a natural genetic mutation.

Peaches and nectarines both originated in China and were brought to America by the Spaniards in the 16th century. Nowadays, approximately 60 percent of peaches and 95 percent of nectarines consumed in the U.S. are grown in California.

Peaches and nectarines contain cancer-fighting phytochemicals such as alpha and beta-carotene. A recent study that followed almost 76,000 women for up to 24 years found that those who ate at least two servings per week of peaches or nectarines had a 41 percent lower risk of developing post-menopausal ER- breast cancer than those who didn't.[21] Another study found that treating estrogen-dependent breast cancer cells with peach and plum extracts killed the cancer cells without harming normal cells.[23]

And a study published in the *Journal of Medicinal Food* in 2009 found that the peels and flesh of peaches both contain a particular antioxidant—chlorogenic acid—that scavenges free radicals and may deter diseases such as cancer.[24]

In addition to preventing cancer, eating peaches and nectarines may reduce the risk of cardiovascular disease and fight metabolic syndrome, which is a precursor to diabetes and a host of other significant health issues. These fruits are good sources of fiber, vitamins C and A, and minerals such as potassium.

Eat peaches and nectarines during the summer when in season. For both fruits, buying organic is definitely best; peaches and nectarines both frequent the EWG's "Dirty Dozen" list.

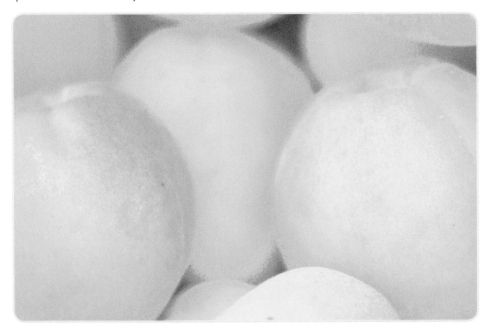

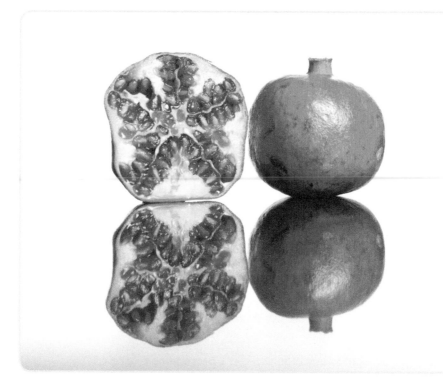

Praise Pomegranate

Pomegranates have been around since ancient times. Some Bible scholars even believe it to be the original forbidden fruit in the Garden of Eden. Although native to Iran, the majority of pomegranates sold in the U.S. are grown in California today.

The pomegranate can be a powerful weapon in your fight against breast cancer! Research has identified six chemicals in the pomegranate that suppress aromatase, an enzyme used by breast cancer cells to produce estrogen.[25] Since approximately 70 percent of breast cancers need estrogen to grow, when you can suppress that enzyme, you may be able to suppress breast cancer itself.

Another recent study showed that a combination of three specific components of pomegranate juice keep cancer cells together, thus decreasing their ability to wander off and wreak havoc elsewhere.

This same study found that pomegranate juice and its components also inhibit the spread of breast cancer cells to the bone.[26] In general, cancer becomes dangerous and deadly when it begins to spread or metastasize.

Pomegranate benefits don't end at cancer fighting. This fruit is also high in antioxidants and rich in fiber, folate, and vitamins B5, C, E, and K as well as calcium, copper, potassium, and manganese. Pomegranates and their juice have been linked to lowering blood pressure and preventing heart disease in people with diabetes.

Lift Safely

To Juice or Not to Juice

Normally, most nutrition experts don't recommend drinking fruit juice; it can have as much sugar as soda with negligible nutritional benefits.

However, pomegranate juice could be the exception. Some research has shown that the sugars in pomegranate juice do not spike your blood sugar. That said, drink it in moderation and follow these simple tips to getting the most out of your pomegranate juice:

- An old joke seen on t-shirts at mountain resorts features the green beginner circle atop the words "I suck." But there's no beginner level when it comes to pomegranate juice. *That* t-shirt should say, "Go big or go home." Remember, juice with added sugar, color, or flavor is not actually pomegranate juice. "It sucks."

- You can buy pomegranate juice from concentrate that has only added water; it's less expensive than pure pomegranate juice. (A good, reasonably priced brand is Pom Wonderful.)

- ◆ Ideally, you want to buy organic, 100% pomegranate juice not from concentrate. However, expect to pay an arm and a leg for it. To get your greatest benefit, combine small amounts in a smoothie with organic soymilk. In fact, a compound in soy known as genistein has been shown to boost the cancer-fighting powers of pomegranate.[27]

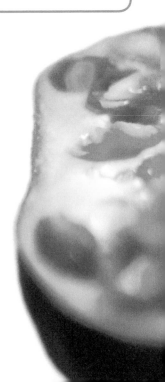

Discovery Center
Deseeding a Pomegranate

Reluctant to spend 30 minutes deseeding a pomegranate and end up with your kitchen walls looking like a scene from the CSI television show? The following fool-proof method can be done in less than a minute:

- ✿ To loosen the seeds, firmly press the pomegranate into the countertop or cutting board with your hands and roll it around.

- ✿ Think of the cluster at the top as the North Pole and cut the pomegranate in half around what would be its equator.

- ✿ Hold each half over a large bowl and whack on the pomegranate's back with a large wooden or metal spoon. Be careful not to hit your hand! Watch the seeds fall into the bowl.

- ✿ Sprinkle its seeds on salads, smoothies, yogurt, ice cream, or whatever suits your fancy.

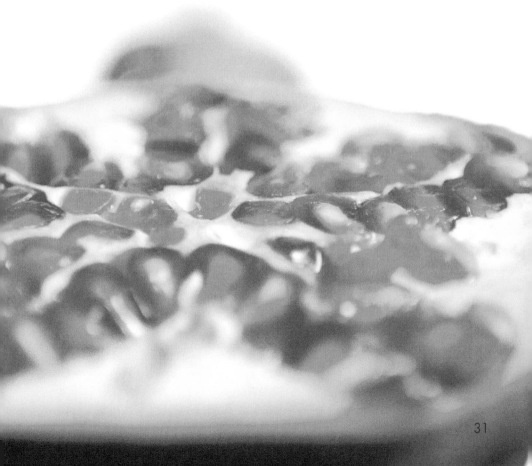

Herbs and Spices

No, "herbs" aren't the geeky accountants in your neighborhood. And "spices"; well, for centuries they've been so highly prized, Christopher Columbus sailed the seas in search of them.

Both herbs and spices are an extremely valuable weapon in your cancer-fighting arsenal. Unfortunately, many unsavory ingredients—lead, artificial colors, insects, rodent hairs, etc.—have been found in spices. In addition, herbs are often loaded with pesticide residue. For both spices and herbs, always buy high-quality and/or organic products from a company you trust.

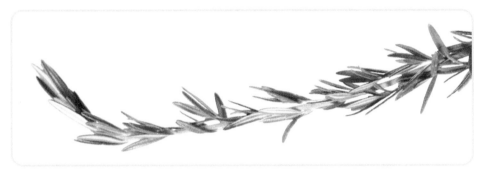

Go for Ginger

Ginger is widely recognized for its ability to treat gastro-intestinal distress. However, ginger's health benefits don't stop there. This potent anti-inflammatory spice is one of the world's oldest medicinal foods. In fact, studies have linked ginger to more than 100 different health benefits.

One particular benefit is ginger's ability to fight breast cancer. As one study showed, a compound in ginger known as [6]-gingerol inhibits cell adhesion, invasion, motility, and activities of certain human breast cancer cell lines. That indicates ginger stops the metastasis or spread of breast cancer![28]

Another study showed that ginger suppressed the growth and colony formation of breast cancer cells without harming normal cells.[29]

In addition to breast cancer, several studies have shown ginger to be effective against colon and ovarian cancers as well as others. It's also been called a "miracle" cure for chemotherapy-induced vomiting.[30]

So what are you waiting for? Add some ginger spice to your life! You'll find ginger widely available as a condiment in Japanese restaurants. At home, add grated or sliced ginger to fresh juices, stir fries, soups, and baked goods. You can even make your own ginger tea.

Quick Eats

Homemade Ginger Tea

This easy-to-make, inexpensive tea is a great way to add ginger to your diet:

- ✿ 2 tbsp peeled and freshly grated or sliced ginger
- ✿ 2 cups water

Put water and ginger in a saucepan and bring to a boil. Reduce heat and simmer for 15-20 minutes. Strain the mixture into a cup. Add lemon juice, raw honey, agave nectar, or other natural sweetener to taste.

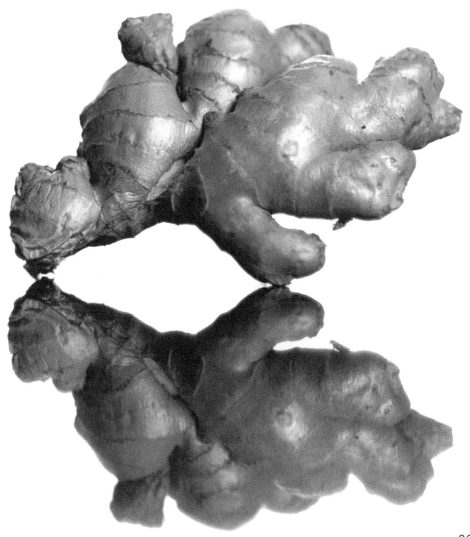

33

⑫ Pine for Parsley

Like celery, parsley is a member of the Apiaceae family. Believed to have originated in the Mediterranean region, it has been grown for medicinal purposes for more than 2,000 years. In the 17th century, European colonists brought parsley to America.

One of the most commonly grown herbs, parsley flourishes in a wide variety of conditions and is popular in herb gardens across the U.S.

Like celery, parsley contains the antioxidant apigenin. Research has shown that this substance shrank a type of tumor caused by a particularly deadly, fast-growing human breast cancer cell, with no toxic side effects.[7]

In addition to apigenin, parsley provides many more antioxidants; more than your vitamin K requirements for the day; vitamins A and C; folate; and minerals such as calcium, iron, manganese, magnesium, and potassium. An anti-inflammatory, parsley may lower blood pressure and helps the kidneys (unless you already have kidney or gall bladder problems, in which case it's best to avoid eating parsley).

Be sure to include plenty o' parsley in your diet. It can be added to casseroles, soups, stews, or other cooked dishes; also eat it raw in salads and fresh green juices.

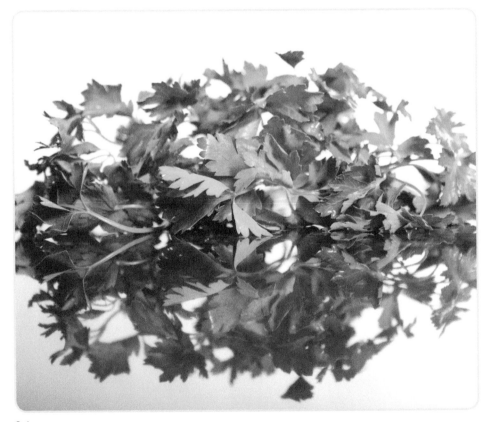

Parsley Almond Vegan Pesto

This super scrumptious pesto will have you gobbling up parsley in no time:

- 1 cup Italian flat leaf parsley
- 1 tbsp sautéed garlic and onion
- ½ cup raw almonds
- ¼ cup olive oil
- ¼ cup water
- ½ tsp salt
- ½ tsp pepper
- ½ lemon (juiced)

Combine all ingredients in a food processor and blend until smooth. Use in pasta or cooked quinoa, or as a delicious spread on sandwiches.

Thanks to Chef Marc Rouse from FOOD! by Marc *in Avon, CO for providing this amazing recipe.*

Reach for Rosemary

Rosemary is a member of the mint family. Native to the Mediterranean region, this herb was used in ancient times as the universal symbol of remembrance for those who passed away. It's also used to symbolize fidelity and remembrance during wedding ceremonies. Today, rosemary is grown in temperate regions throughout the world.

Rosemary contains a substance called carnosol, shown to detoxify substances that can initiate the breast-cancer process.[31] Research has also shown that rosemary suppresses the development of tumors not only in the breast but in the colon, liver, and stomach. It also affects melanoma and leukemia cells.[32]

Yet another study showed that rosemary stimulates a liver enzyme that inactivates estrogen hormones—important because excessive estrogen hormones in women can contribute to the growth of breast cancer cells.[33]

In addition, rosemary is anti-inflammatory, antiviral, antimicrobial, antibacterial, and an antioxidant. This amazing herb contains fiber, iron, and calcium. It can also stimulate your immune system, increase circulation, improve digestion, enhance memory, protect your eyes from macular degeneration, and protect the brain from aging and free-radical damage. It's even believed to stimulate hair growth.

Use fresh or dried rosemary in Mediterranean or Italian dishes, soups, salads, breads, and even desserts.

Safer Cooking With Rosemary

Cooking animal protein (meat, poultry, fish) at high temperatures causes the formation of chemical compounds called heterocyclic amines (HCAs). These compounds are linked to the formation of some cancers.

In addition, cooking carbohydrate-rich foods at high temperatures causes the formation of acrylamides (a neurotoxic chemical), which may be linked to cancer.

The good news is that marinating your meat, poultry, or fish in a sauce that contains rosemary has been shown to significantly decrease the number of HCAs formed. Adding rosemary to carbohydrate-rich foods such as bread can significantly reduce the number of acrylamides formed when cooked at high temperatures.

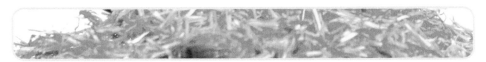

Save for Saffron

Saffron, the most expensive spice in the world, comes from the purple crocus flower. One acre of the plant yields only one pound of this spice.

Saffron is grown primarily in the Mediterranean region and India, with Spain being the top producer in the world. Cleopatra is rumored to have been a big fan of saffron; she bathed in it to "enhance" her lovemaking.

Saffron contains a carotenoid called crocetin as well as various crocins that have been shown to inhibit the growth of breast cancer cells. One study noted that crocetin also inhibited the degree of invasiveness of a highly invasive type of breast cancer cell.[34]

In addition to inhibiting breast cancer, studies indicate saffron extract can inhibit the growth of skin, liver, colorectal, and leukemia cancer cells. It can act as an antidepressant and help symptoms of PMS.

Although saffron is expensive, you only need a few threads of it to color and flavor your meals. Add it to eggs, pasta or rice dishes, risotto, soups or broths, even desserts—anything that strikes you.

Unmarked Obstacles

Saffron may be toxic at high doses, so stick to using it in spice form rather than extracts or pills.

15 Try Turmeric

Turmeric, a relative of ginger, is a spice grown in India and certain regions of Asia. For centuries, turmeric has been used for medicinal purposes in Chinese medicine and Indian Ayurvedic medicine. Used in both Indian and Asian cooking, it's an ingredient in a common mix of spices known as curry.

Turmeric contains an antioxidant called curcumin, which has been shown in laboratory studies to inhibit several types of cancer cells. In one study, researchers at the University of Texas MD Anderson Cancer Center found that curcumin reduces the expression of a particular molecule in aggressive breast cancer cells that makes the disease more deadly. These aggressive cells are responsible for the spread of the disease to other parts of the body, which means curcumin could potentially slow or halt the spread of the disease.[35]

In addition, another study showed that a combination of curcumin and piperine (the compound that makes both black and white pepper hot) could eliminate breast cancer stem cells without damaging healthy tissue.[36] Why is this important? Think of breast cancer stem cells as terrorist sleeper cells; they lay low to avoid detection and treatment, only to later resurface, form new colonies of cells, and wreak havoc on the body.

Turmeric's magic isn't limited to cancer. A potent anti-inflammatory and cell protectant, this spice may lower LDL (bad) cholesterol, reduce arthritis symptoms, treat autoimmune disorders, protect against liver damage, and prevent Alzheimer's disease. In fact, elderly villagers in India have the lowest Alzheimer's rates in the world—believed to be due to the high amounts of turmeric in their diet.

Strive to eat turmeric every day. Add turmeric to your diet by mixing it in with scrambled or sprinkling it on fried or poached eggs. Dust it on cooked vegetables or add to soups, chili, or other dishes. You can add a small amount (about an eighth of a teaspoon) of turmeric to smoothies. You won't even taste it!

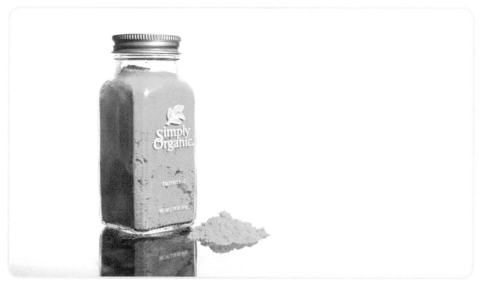

Pumpkin Smoothie

This delicious smoothie is a great way to add healthy seeds and turmeric to your diet.

- 1 cup unsweetened almond milk
- 1 frozen banana, broken into 1-inch pieces
- 1 tbsp ground flax seeds
- 1 tbsp chia seeds
- 1 scoop vegan vanilla protein powder
- 1 tsp pure maple syrup
- ½ cup pumpkin puree
- ¼ tsp cinnamon
- ⅛ tsp turmeric

Blend for about one minute in a Vitamix or other powerful blender. Top with extra treats like cacao nibs, dried mulberries, or coconut flakes.

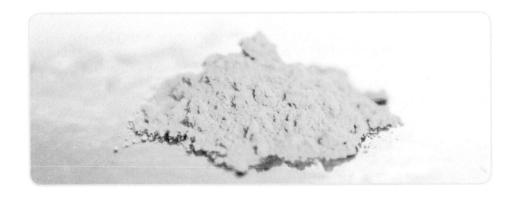

Turmeric Tips

Turmeric, along with rosemary, garlic, sage, and cherries, can reduce the carcinogenic chemicals that form in barbecued, broiled, or fried meat.

Whenever you're using turmeric, make sure to include black pepper. This combination drastically increases the body's absorption of the nutrients.

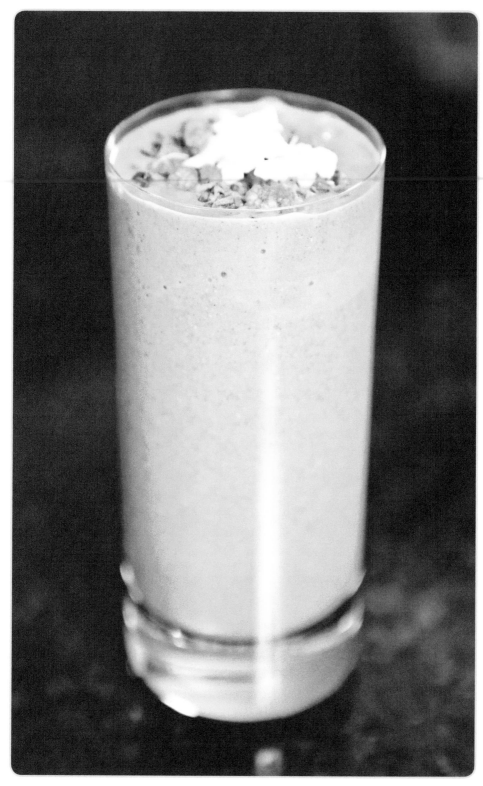

Nuts, Seeds, and Beans

16 Dig Dark Chocolate

You'll love me for this one! Good news about chocolate (cacao) is all over the place these days. It seems you can't open a magazine or turn on TV without hearing about its benefits.

Cacao originated in Central America where the Mayans and Aztecs used it for centuries, both as food and currency. Christopher Columbus first introduced cacao to Europe early in the 16th century. Over the next century or so, it became quite popular in Spain, France, Germany, and Italy. Chocolate wasn't produced in America until the mid-18th century.[37]

What makes cacao good for you? It's loaded with antioxidants called flavanols. Along with coffee (another bean), it's also one of the best sources of antioxidants on the planet. The antioxidants in dark chocolate have been shown to fight cell damage that may lead to tumor growth. One study indicated a substance in cocoa deactivated certain proteins in breast cancer cells, which prevented them from dividing further.[38]

Plus, here's a small taste (pun intended) of even more benefits. Chocolate:

❀ Works as an antidepressant and improves mood (duh!),

❀ Raises one's libido (huh?!),

❀ Raises HDL cholesterol (the good stuff),

❀ Lowers blood sugar,

❀ Improves brain function, and

❀ May lower blood pressure.

In addition to antioxidants, you'll find cacao chock full of nutrients including fiber, potassium, magnesium, manganese, copper, zinc, selenium, and phosphorus. This nutritional powerhouse has been linked with a healthy heart and brain, improved cholesterol profile, and even lower blood pressure.

Go for the good stuff; you're worth it! For more cacao and less sugar, fat, and who knows what else, it's best to buy chocolate that's at least 70% cacao, organic, and fairly traded. The mass-produced "cheap" stuff doesn't cut it. In fact, many of these kinds of chocolate contain little or no actual cacao.

At 12 calories per tablespoon, unsweetened organic cocoa powder is one of the best ways to get the health benefits of cacao. So add it to your smoothies, oatmeal, yogurt, and other foods.

Remember, moderation—about one ounce a day—is key, even with the highest-quality chocolate.

Discovery Center
The 3 C's of Chocolate

When talkin' chocolate, these three words are often tossed around: cacao, cocoa, and chocolate. What's the difference?

Cacao is the actual bean that comes from the cacao tree. It grows inside a large pod on the trunk and limbs of this tree.

Cocoa is the name for the cacao bean after it has been processed, which typically involves fermenting, drying, cleaning, and roasting.

Chocolate is cocoa after the addition of fat and sugar.

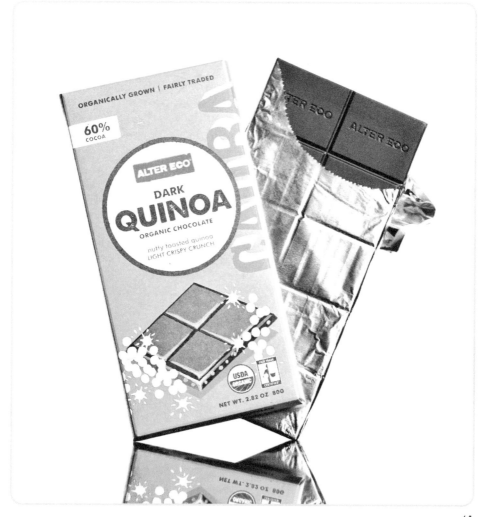

⑰ Feast on Flax

Did you know linen is made from the flax plant? Flax, a flowering plant grown for both its seed and its stalk, is used to make textile fibers.

The flax plant, which originated in the Mediterranean region, was one of the first crops domesticated by man. After being brought to America by European colonists, it was used for clothing fiber, paint, printing ink, animal feed, and other things before becoming almost extinct in the U.S. in the 1940s. After its resurgence in popularity, most flax is now grown domestically in North Dakota or Minnesota.

The key beneficial anti-cancer substances in flax are *lignans*, which are antioxidants that studies show may slow cell growth. Lignans also function as anti-estrogens or weak estrogens and may actually block the effects of estrogen in some tissues, thus reducing the risk of some hormone-associated cancers.[39]

A recent meta-analysis on the effects of flax seeds on breast cancer showed they *increase* apoptosis within tumors and *decrease* breast cancer growth. The study indicated that flax can decrease HER2/neu expression. (Over expression of the HER2/neu gene leads to the development and progression of certain aggressive forms of the disease.)

Overall, this meta-analysis showed that consumption of flax seeds decreased the risk of developing a first breast cancer by 18 percent and lowered the mortality rate of those with the disease by 31 percent. Better mental health among breast cancer patients has also been noted.[40]

In addition to lignans, flax seeds are rich in beneficial omega-3 fatty acids and fiber, plus they contain important minerals such as manganese, magnesium phosphorus, and copper. Flax seeds have been shown to reduce inflammation, aid the cardiovascular system, reduce oxidative stress, and improve cholesterol ratios.

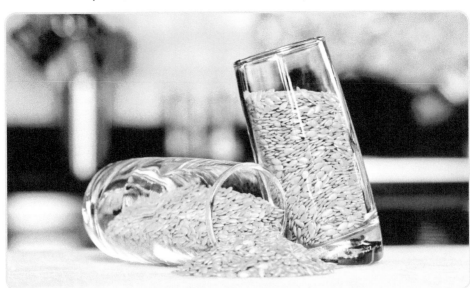

Adding flax seeds to your diet is easy! Put flax seeds in smoothies, use them in baking, and sprinkle them on cereal, oatmeal, or salads. You can even replace eggs in baking with flax. One tablespoon of ground flax in one-quarter cup of water equals one egg.

Unmarked Obstacles
Facts About Flax

Unground flax seeds *cannot* be digested; they'll pass right through you without imparting any of their wonderful benefits. So be sure to grind flax seeds before eating them.

In addition, flax seeds go rancid quite easily, so store them in the refrigerator or freezer for maximum benefit.

Flax seeds may interfere with the absorption of some medications or supplements, so wait one hour or more after eating flax seeds before taking them.

Suggestion: Skip using flax oil. It contains none of the fiber and few of the beneficial lignans that flax seeds have.

 ## Long for Legumes

Beans, peas, lentils, and peanuts are in a class of vegetables known as legumes. Legumes have a long and storied history, with certain types cultivated as far back as 20,000 years. Some legumes are native to the Mediterranean region, some to Asia, and still others come from South and Central America where they've been staples of the Incan and Aztec diets.

Beans and lentils have shown a lot of promise in fighting breast cancer. The Nurses Health Study II followed more than 90,000 women over eight years. It found that women who ate beans or lentils at least two times a week had a 24 percent lower risk of developing breast cancer than those who ate them once a month or less.[41]

Another study performed on laboratory mice showed that eating dried beans inhibited the development of breast cancer and caused cells to undergo apoptosis.[42]

Beans and lentils don't only fight breast cancer. Eating beans is linked with a lower risk of diabetes, heart disease, and certain other types of cancer. They are high in fiber, low in calories, and contain no cholesterol. Overall, you'll find beans loaded with antioxidants, folate, B vitamins, copper, iron, magnesium, manganese, phosphorus, and potassium. Eat a variety to ensure you get all of these nutrients.

Low cost is one of their best benefits. Dried organic beans and lentils can be found in the bulk section of a natural foods store for only a couple dollars per pound. Use them to replace meat in your meals several times a week. You can also extend the meat in a dish like chili or tacos by adding beans, thus making it healthier *and* less expensive.

Discovery Center
A Word About Soy

Soy, a type of bean, is one of the most controversial topics in nutrition. The Internet is full of discussions about the "dangers" of soy, with some calling it "toxic." Breast cancer survivors are frequently told to avoid it.

But is soy really dangerous?

Some believe soy should be avoided because it contains phytoestrogens (naturally occurring plant estrogens), which behave like a weak estrogen in the body. This appears troubling because, when estrogen meets an estrogen receptor in a breast cell, breast cancer can occur.

However, these phytoestrogens are nowhere nearly as strong as human estrogen.

Plus they show anti-estrogen effects. That means when these weak estrogens bind to an estrogen receptor, they block more potent natural estrogens. Phytoestrogens also block the formation of estrogens in fat tissue, and they are anti-inflammatory and anti-oxidant. Both of these factors can reduce cancer growth.[43]

In addition, a 2010 study showed that post-menopausal Chinese estrogen and progesterone receptor positive breast cancer survivors who ate the most soy isoflavones had a 33 percent lower chance of recurrence than those who ate less than 15 mg per day. (These survivors ate more than 42 mg a day or the equivalent of one-half cup of tofu.) [44]

Soy can be difficult for some to digest and is one of the most common food sensitivities. If that describes you but you'd still enjoy having soy occasionally, try fermented soy products such as tempeh, miso, natto, and naturally fermented soy sauce. The fermentation process makes foods such as soy (and dairy) easier to digest.

Lastly, take these precautions when eating soy:

- Buy organic. Approximately 90 percent of the soy grown in the U.S. is genetically modified. Conventional soy is also high in pesticide residue.

- Avoid fake meats, cheeses, ice creams, etc. that contain isolated soy proteins, or eat them in extreme moderation. These do not have the same protective qualities as whole soy foods and may actually be dangerous.

- Stick with less processed soy foods like edamame, tofu, and soy milk with only a few ingredients. (WestSoy is a good brand.) Avoid soy milks that contain carrageenan, a substance derived from seaweed that some experts believe may be carcinogenic.

- Do not take soy supplements. Study results regarding benefits are mixed and they may actually be harmful.

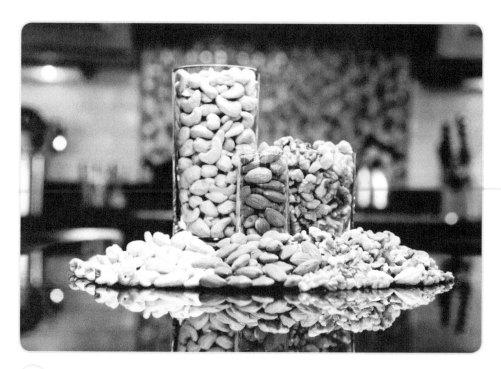

Nosh on Nuts

Many of the plants we call nuts aren't actually nuts. Several are actually seeds from the fruit of certain trees and others are technically drupes—that is, fleshy fruits that contain a seed. Peanuts, despite the name, are actually legumes in the same family as beans and peas. Hazelnuts and chestnuts are two of the more commonly eaten "true" nuts. These plants are native to regions all over the world, depending on the type. Of the most common varieties, only pecans are native to North America.

Back in the low-fat diet craze (glad those days are over!), lots of folks avoided nuts because of their fat and calories. Today, we know better. Nuts are supremely healthful and have even shown promise in preventing cancer.

One recent study showed that girls aged 9 to 15 who ate a daily serving of vegetable fat from foods such as peanuts and nuts had a lower risk of developing benign breast disease (BBD) by age 30 than those who didn't eat them. In girls with a family history of breast cancer, the risk of developing BBD was significantly lower with the consumption of these foods.[45]

Note: While BBD is not cancerous itself, it does raise the risk of developing breast cancer later in life.

Walnuts in particular have shown promise in stopping breast cancer in its tracks. First, they contain several nutrients such as omega-3 fatty acids, antioxidants, and other phytonutrients that individually have been shown to slow cancer growth. In addition, one laboratory study found a significant reduction in the incidence, number, and size of breast tumors in the mice that were fed walnuts.[46]

The wonder of nuts doesn't stop at cancer prevention. An anti-inflammatory, they've been shown to reduce LDL (bad) cholesterol, lower the risk of heart disease, stabilize blood sugar (by slowing down digestion), and even help maintain a healthy weight. Nuts provide protein, fiber, folate, vitamins A, B, D, and E, and important minerals such as calcium, copper, manganese, magnesium, phosphorus, potassium, selenium, and zinc.

Choosing a variety of nuts ensures you take in all of these nutrients. And when it comes to eating nuts, raw is best. Nuts contain delicate oils that get damaged by heating, which leads to the creation of free radicals in your body. In addition, roasted nuts can be loaded with salt or even sugar. For the occasional treat of roasted nuts, go for the dry roasted kind without added oils or sugar.

Eat about one-quarter cup (the equivalent of one small handful) of nuts each day. Sprinkle them on hot or cold cereals, smoothies, and salads, or eat as a snack. You can also boost the protein in your smoothies or pureed soups by adding nuts.

Quick Eats
Homemade Vanilla Almond Milk

Unfortunately, many commercial non-dairy types of milk are loaded with sugar and other additives. Once you make your own almond milk, you won't want to go back to the store-bought variety.

- 1 cup almonds, soaked in water overnight or for several hours
- 4 cups of water
- 2-4 pitted merjool dates (depending on desired sweetness)
- 1 teaspoon vanilla extract
- pinch of sea salt

For plain almond milk, eliminate the last three ingredients.

Place all ingredients in a high-speed blender such as a Vitamix and blend for 1-2 minutes. Strain through a nut bag or cheesecloth, then store in the refrigerator in an airtight glass jar or bottle.

Homemade almond milk will last about five days in the refrigerator.

 Seek Out Seeds

While flaxseeds have their own shout-out, don't ignore other seeds. Like nuts, seeds are an important part of a healthy diet. Some commonly eaten seeds include sunflower, pumpkin, chia, hemp, poppy, and sesame seeds. Depending on their type, seeds are native to regions all over the world.

Like flax seeds, sunflower, pumpkin, sesame, and poppy seeds all contain lignans, an antioxidant that may slow cell growth and prevent estrogen-dependent cancers. Flax seeds are by far the richest source of lignans, though.

In addition, seeds (along with other plant foods such as real whole grains, fruits, and vegetables) are high in phytoestrogens, a naturally occurring chemical found in plants. One study found that women who had the highest intake of phytoestrogens experienced a substantial reduction in breast cancer risk.[47]

Seeds are anti-inflammatory and help maintain healthy cholesterol levels, reduce risk of heart disease and stabilize blood sugar levels. They also contain protein, fiber, omega-3 fatty acids, and are rich in a variety of vitamins and minerals.

Eat one ounce of seeds, or about two tablespoons, at least five times a week. Sprinkle seeds on oatmeal, cereal, smoothies, salads, or simply as a snack. As with nuts, eating them raw is best so you avoid taking in excess salt and damaging delicate oils.

Lift Safely

Digesting Nuts, Seeds, Legumes, and Beans

Raw nuts and seeds as well as legumes, grains, beans, and soy contain substances called phytates—anti-nutrients that can block the absorption of certain important minerals.

Nuts, seeds, and soy also contain another anti-nutrient called trypsin inhibitors, which can stop the body from digesting the food's protein.

For better digestion and absorption of nutrients, soak raw nuts and seeds before consuming them or cooking with them. Soaking disables these anti-nutrients, making them easier to digest and allowing your body to better absorb the nutrients. If possible, soak these foods overnight or at least several hours before cooking or eating them.

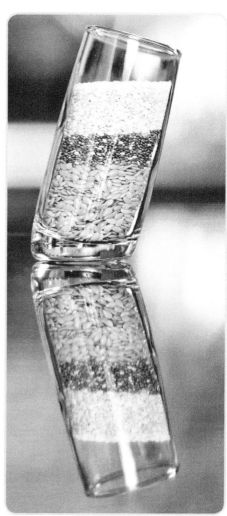

Last But Not Least...

㉑ Devour Vitamin D

Vitamin D, commonly called the "sunshine vitamin," is actually a hormone. It's produced by the body when UVB rays hit unprotected skin, causing cholesterol on the skin to turn into vitamin D3.

To date, the results of studies regarding vitamin D and cancer have varied, with some being inconclusive. However, many studies have shown an association between decreased risk of breast cancer and increased blood levels of vitamin D.

One study conducted by prominent vitamin D researchers showed that women with levels above 52 ng/ml (levels of 32-100 are considered normal) experience half of the breast cancer rate as women who have levels of less than 13 ng/ml.[48] In addition, some of these same researchers determined that out of the approximately 230,000 new cases of breast cancer each year, increased blood levels of 52 ng/ml could prevent about 58,000 of these cases.[49]

If that doesn't grab you, vitamin D has also been shown to protect against other cancers, strengthen the bones, boost the immune system, protect against certain autoimmune diseases (such as multiple sclerosis), and reduce the chance of heart disease.

Insist that your doctor test your vitamin D level at your next checkup. Optimal blood levels of vitamin D fall between 50 and 70 ng/ml. Over 32 is considered "normal" but not optimal for disease prevention. If you have cancer or heart disease, levels of 70 to 100 ng/ml may be more appropriate; however, you should not exceed levels of 100 ng/ml.[50] The best test for checking blood levels is the 25(OH)D, also known as 25-hydroxyvitamin D.

The current government recommendation for Vitamin D is 600 IU (international units) for people aged 1 through 70 and 800 IU for those 71 and above. However, many experts recommend supplementing with 1,000 to 2,000 IU a day—perhaps even more, especially during the winter months.

Lift Safely
D2 or D3 – Which is Better?

If you plan to supplement with vitamin D, make sure the product contains D3 and not D2. Vitamin D3 is the type made by our bodies when the skin gets hit with UVB rays. Our bodies use it much better than D2, which is made by plants exposed to ultraviolet light.

Be careful. Many prescription and supplement forms of D as well as most fortified foods contain D2.

Get Your D On

By far, your best way to obtain vitamin D is from the sun. Did you know that a fair-skinned person can produce approximately 10,000 IU of D3 in just 10 minutes of unprotected mid-day sun? The darker your skin, the more time you'll need.

Yet, in many parts of the country, it's impossible for your body to produce vitamin D during the winter months. North of Atlanta or Los Angeles, you could lay out in the sun naked all the livelong day and not produce any vitamin D during the winter. With the sun being low in the sky, its angle won't allow the UVB rays to penetrate the atmosphere.

It's also difficult to get adequate vitamin D from diet alone; few foods contain D and those that do contain very low levels. What are the best food sources of vitamin D? Cod liver oil, wild salmon, and certain other fatty fish.

Note: Wild salmon contains more than four times the amount of vitamin D as farmed salmon. Go wild!

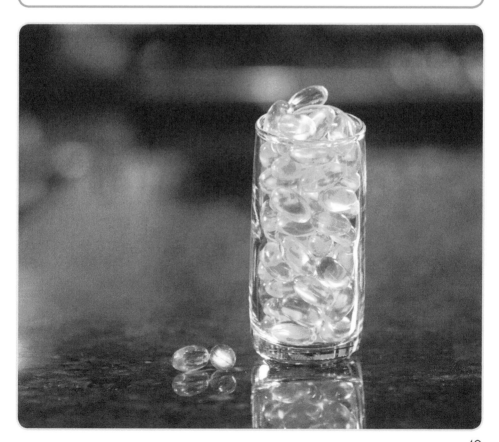

Feed on Fermented Foods

Humans have been fermenting foods since ancient times. During the fermentation process, the food is exposed to bacteria and yeasts under anaerobic (without oxygen) conditions, with the carbohydrates in the food converting to alcohols or organic acids.

Fermentation preserves food without cooking it and destroying its beneficial enzymes, bacteria, and other nutrients. Common fermented foods are yogurt (including coconut milk yogurt), certain vinegars, pickles, sauerkraut, kimchi, miso, tempeh, natto, and a newly popular drink called kombucha.

If you've had any of these, you know that fermented foods can sometimes have a funky taste or smell. Still, their health benefits outweigh any funkiness. That includes a reduction in the risk of breast cancer. For example, one study of Japanese women showed that those who ate more of a fermented soy product called miso had a 54 percent lower risk of developing the disease than those who didn't.[51]

In addition to potentially reducing your risk of breast cancer, fermented foods improve digestion. This allows you to absorb more of the vitamins and minerals in the food you eat. They also help you maintain a healthy gut by introducing probiotics ("good" bacteria) and digestive enzymes. *These enzymes are crucial because as much as 80 percent of your immune system cells are located in your gut.*

Be selective when choosing your fermented foods. For example, while pickles can be a fermented food, not all pickles are created equal. Pickles that sit on the store shelf (rather than in the refrigerated section) have been pasteurized and aren't fermented. To ensure food is fermented, make your own or look for the words "live cultures" on the packaging at the store.

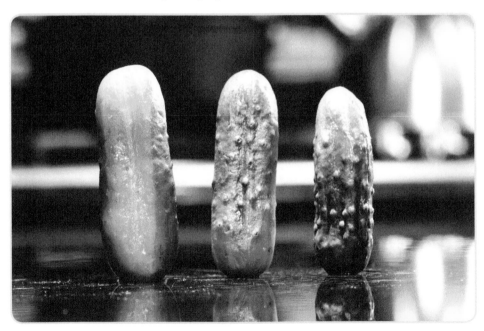

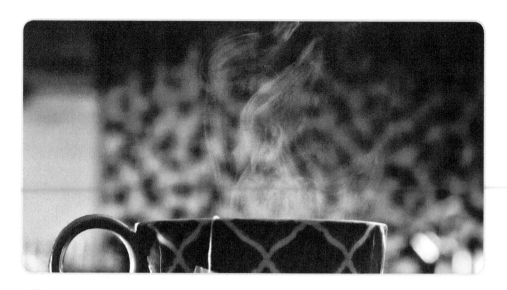

23 Guzzle Green Tea

Green tea originated in Asia and has been drunk by the Chinese and Japanese for thousands of years. It's made from young tea leaves briefly steamed to stop the oxidation process that would normally turn them black.

While tea plants can only grow in warm climates, green tea is enjoyed all over the world, partly because of its amazing health benefits. It contains compounds called polyphenols, a type of antioxidant. One of its main polyphenols is a compound called epigallocatechin-3-gallate, commonly referred to as EGCG. Because green tea undergoes minimal processing, many of these polyphenols are retained.

Studies to date regarding the effects of green tea on cancer have been inconclusive or conflicting. However, some laboratory and animal studies have shown that EGCG and other polyphenols in green tea may prevent cancer from forming, while also limiting the growth and migration of breast cancer cells.[52]

In addition, a 2006 meta-analysis that reviewed the results of 13 studies involving participants from eight countries found that women who drank the most green tea had a lower risk of breast cancer than those who drank the least.[53]

Note: Overall breast cancer rates are lower in countries such as Japan where people drink green tea regularly.

Aside from its possible cancer-fighting effects, green tea has been shown to reduce the risk of certain other types of cancer as well as lower blood pressure and total cholesterol. It's known to raise good cholesterol, control blood sugar levels, and even blast belly fat.

The recommended amount of green tea to drink is three to four cups a day. If that seems unrealistic, consider supplementing what you drink with a high-quality green tea extract. Be sure to consult with your natural health practitioner first.

Get the Most From Your Tea

To get the most nutrients from your tea, add a squeeze of lemon. The vitamin C in a small amount of lemon juice will help your body absorb more of the tea's antioxidants. And ditch both the milk *and* soymilk. The proteins in both can bind to the antioxidants in tea and neutralize them.

Willing to "green light" some green tea? Then choose quality ingredients. Use this guide to hit an expert level as quickly as possible:

- Avoid cheap grocery store or massed-produced national brands. Many brands found in supermarkets do not contain much actual green tea. Also, run from any tea containing artificial flavors or colors, soy lecithin, or other strange ingredients. Your lovely cup of morning tea has just become a highly processed food.

- Buy organic. Most tea is sprayed liberally with pesticides and doesn't get washed before being bagged and sold to you. These pesticides harm both you and the farmer who grew the tea leafs. Avoid vague-sounding "natural flavors" wording. These flavors may not come from sources you'd expect.

- Pay attention to packaging. Many so-called "wellness" or "premium" brands package their teas in bags made of plastic or genetically modified substances. Heating plastic to a temperature even below boiling point can potentially cause harmful chemicals to leach into your tea. Organic loose leaf tea is your best option.

24 Honor Omega 3s

Omega-3 fatty acids are a group of three fats – ALA, DHA, and EPA. These fats are considered *essential*, meaning they're needed to survive, yet our bodies cannot produce them on their own. Therefore, we must get these fats from our diet.

Many experts say the most important of these three fats are DHAs and EPAs found in certain fish, algae, and krill (tiny, shrimp-like crustaceans). ALAs—present in flaxseeds, chia seeds, walnuts, and certain other plants—are the precursor to DHAs and EPAs.

Some researchers contend that the body does a poor job of converting ALAs to the other two fats. However, as with many topics in nutrition, this is widely debated.

Some evidence exists that omega-3s may help prevent breast cancer. One meta-analysis reviewed the results of 26 studies including almost 900,000 participants and 21,000 cases of breast cancer. It showed a 14 percent reduction in risk for women who got their omega-3s from marine sources.[54] In addition, DHA has been shown to induce apoptosis in triple-negative breast cancer cells.[55] Lastly, one laboratory study showed that omega-3s may help prevent the spread of breast cancer.[56]

In addition to potentially lowering your risk of breast cancer, omega-3s have been linked to preventing sudden cardiac death. They are also linked to lower triglycerides, lower blood pressure, better cholesterol profile, reduced arthritis symptoms, improved autoimmune disease symptoms, help with depression, and many more benefits.

While fatty fish such as salmon, mackerel, and tuna are great sources of omega-3s, the issues of overfishing and environmental toxins can't be ignored. When it comes to toxins such as mercury, the smaller the fish, the less mercury will have accumulated in its body. Therefore, turning to sources such as sardines, anchovies, and krill are a good way to get your omega-3s.

Note: If you are vegan, plant sources of ALAs may not give you all the omega-3s you need due to the potentially poor conversion of ALA to DHA and EPA. However, algae sources are a good way to obtain DHA and EPA.

Aim to take in at least 500 mg of combined DHA and EPA a day. Whichever source you choose—fish or algae—purchase the best quality you can find to protect both your body and the earth from environmental toxins.

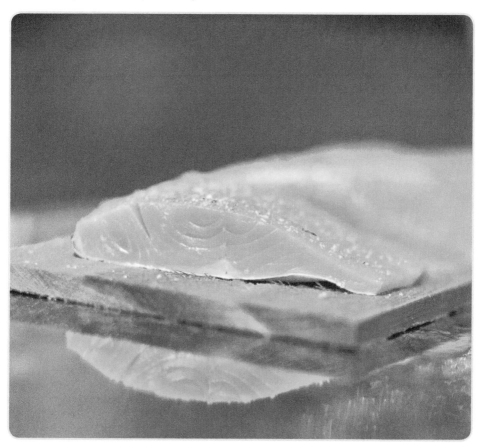

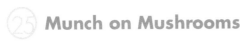

Munch on Mushrooms

Humans have been eating mushrooms for thousands of years. In ancient Egypt, the pharaohs believed eating mushrooms would make them immortal and made them illegal for commoners to eat.

The cultivation of mushrooms began in Europe during the 17th century but didn't begin in America until the late 1800s. A town in southeastern Pennsylvania called Kennett Square had the first mushroom farm in America. Interestingly, about half of the mushrooms grown in the U.S. today come from that same small town.

Mushrooms are one of the most potent anti-cancer foods known. In fact, they are such powerful cancer-fighters that studies say only *one mushroom a day* may decrease your breast cancer risk by 60+ percent.[57]

Just how do mushrooms work against breast cancer? Even when the ovaries are producing little to no estrogen (as in post-menopausal women), breast cancer cells can make estrogen using an enzyme called aromatase. Many of the drugs used today for estrogen positive breast cancer are, in fact, aromatase inhibitors. Mushrooms contain natural aromatase inhibitors, which may help decrease blood estrogen levels and slow breast cancer growth.

In addition to having anti-cancer properties, mushrooms are antioxidant, anti-inflammatory, and antiviral, while enhancing the immune system. Certain mushrooms—maitakes, shiitakes, and criminis—are believed to protect against cardiovascular disease.

Remember, eating even one mushroom a day can have incredible benefits. All types of mushrooms protect against cancer.

Make any of these mushrooms a cornerstone of your anti-cancer diet: white button, crimini, Portobello, shitake, maitake, chanterelles, oyster mushrooms, and others. Add them to pasta and rice dishes, risotto, soups, stews, pizza, or any cooked dish your heart desires.

Unmarked Obstacles
Should You Eat Raw Mushrooms?

No. Never eat raw mushrooms, which are difficult to digest. In fact, many varieties will make you downright sick if eaten raw. Even the white button mushrooms that are commonly served raw at salad bars shouldn't be eaten that way.

Raw mushrooms contain potentially cancer-causing compounds called hydrazines. Heat inactivates most of these compounds so always make sure your mushrooms are well cooked.

In addition, white button and Portobello mushrooms contain a particular hydrazine called agaritine, which is resistant to the effects of heat. So if you want to be extra cautious, avoid or limit your consumption of those varieties.

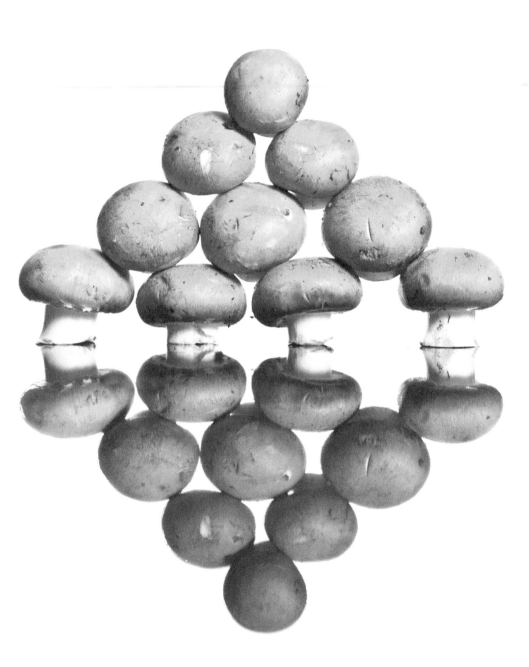

Danger Ahead!

 Abstain From Alcohol

Drastically reducing or eliminating alcohol is one of your most potent weapons in reducing your chances of developing breast cancer. Here's why.

Several studies have shown a very clear link between the consumption of alcohol and a woman's risk of developing breast cancer. One meta-analysis of 53 different studies included more than 58,000 women with invasive breast cancer and over 95,000 women without it. This study found that for each alcoholic drink consumed a day, the relative risk of breast cancer increased by about 7 percent. And consuming two to three alcoholic drinks a day raised a woman's chance of developing breast cancer *by 20 percent!* [58]

In addition, the study concluded that approximately four percent of breast cancers in people in developed countries are caused by the consumption of alcohol. With more than 232,000 cases of invasive breast cancer diagnosed in 2013 as well as over 64,000 cases of DCIS, this equates to in excess of *12,000 preventable cases of breast cancer* in one year alone.

The effects of alcohol seem to be especially detrimental in younger women whose breast cells are rapidly growing. A 2013 study showed that girls and women who drank only one drink a day between their first period and first pregnancy raised their risk of developing breast cancer by 13 percent. Their risk of benign breast disease, which also raises the risk of breast cancer, increased by about 15 percent. [59]

Why does drinking alcohol cause breast cancer? First, alcohol changes the way women metabolize estrogen, which can lead to increased blood estrogen levels. In addition, alcohol consumption can decrease blood levels of folate, which is involved in copying and repairing DNA. If these levels are low, the chances of DNA being copied incorrectly increase. Therefore, if you do drink, get adequate folate in your diet by eating "real" food that includes green vegetables. (See Tip 31 to learn the difference between folate and folic acid.)

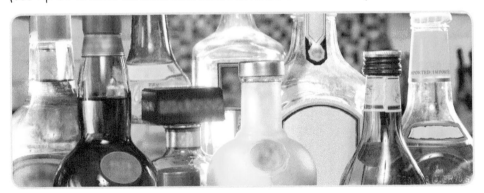

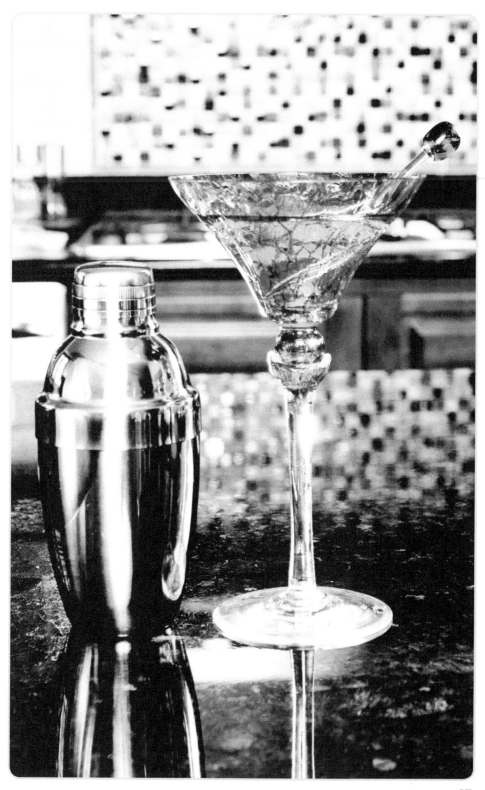

Axe the Artificial Sweeteners

Artificial sweeteners are synthetic sugar substitutes. Common artificial sweeteners include aspartame (with brand names of NutraSweet and Equal), saccharine (Sweet N' Low), and sucralose (Splenda). Watch for others as well. Because these sweeteners can be hundreds to thousands of times sweeter than regular table sugar, the amount needed is far less and contains far fewer calories than sugar.

Truthfully, you'll find the data on artificial sweeteners and cancer all over the map. Regardless, I don't trust synthetic artificial sweeteners; I discourage you from ingesting them under any circumstances. *If a substance comes from a laboratory, your body isn't designed to handle it.*

In addition to possible links to cancer, these sweeteners have been associated with other health problems. Aspartame has been linked to migraine headaches; Splenda contains chlorine, a dangerous carcinogen, and can cause gas, bloating, and diarrhea; saccharine has been shown to cause cancer in laboratory animals. Is drinking that diet soda really worth the risk?

Studies have also shown that eating artificial sweeteners may have the opposite effect of what you'd expect in avoiding weight gain. Because of the disconnection between the taste and the number of calories eaten, they may actually cause you to overeat. Your brain knows you ate *something* sweet, but your body isn't satisfied and craves more.

Artificial sweeteners are also the mark of a highly processed food, so avoid them.

If you crave something sweet, eat fruit or sweet vegetables such as carrots or sweet potatoes.

Discovery Center
What About Stevia?

In the past several years, stevia has become the wonder sweetener of the holistic health crowd. But is that status warranted?

Made from a South American herb, stevia has shown promise as being safe and possibly even beneficial to one's health. However, not all of the information about stevia is positive. As with other artificial sweeteners, it may cause you to overeat. In addition, it has been linked to infertility in rats.

Until more is known, use stevia in moderation and stick with brands that don't use chemicals in their extraction process. Also, read the label and make sure you're actually getting stevia.

Note: One popular brand, *Truvia*, claims to be stevia but is a highly refined product made primarily from sugar alcohols. It contains only a negligible amount of a substance derived from the stevia plant. In 2013, Cargill (the manufacturer of Truvia) settled a proposed class action lawsuit alleging the company misled consumers by marketing Truvia as "natural." Cargill did not admit any liability under the settlement.

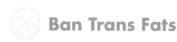 Ban Trans Fats

Trans fatty acids, or trans fats, occur when food manufacturers add hydrogen to an unsaturated fat, such as a vegetable oil. This process changes the oil from one that's liquid at room temperature to one that's solid. The solid fat is more shelf stable and therefore is used to make processed foods last longer on store shelves. Trans fats are frequently found in packaged cookies and crackers, microwave popcorn, coffee creamer, and canned frosting. A small amount of trans fats also occurs naturally in red meats and full fat dairy products.

Man-made trans fats have become one of the worst nutritional nightmares we've been subjected to by the modern food industry—like a heart attack waiting to happen. Several studies have even linked trans fats to the development of breast cancer.

One study from the late 1990s showed that women with the highest levels of trans fatty acids in their adipose (fat) tissue had a 40 percent greater risk of having breast cancer than those with the least amounts of the fat in their tissue.[60] A more recent study showed that women with the highest serum levels of trans fatty acids had a 75 *percent* greater risk of developing invasive breast cancer than those with the lowest serum levels.[61]

Fortunately, the U.S. Food and Drug Administration (FDA) has announced it will require the food industry to gradually phase trans fats out of our food supply. However, because this government agency took so long to act on a problem that's been around for 30+ years, it's unknown how long it will give food companies to complete the phase out.

Until trans fats are completely gone from our food supply, avoid them like the plague.

Unmarked Obstacles

Beware of Hidden Trans Fats

Just because a label says "zero grams trans fats" doesn't mean the product has none.

The FDA allows food companies to say a product has zero grams of trans fats when up to .5 grams are present. That means, given the unrealistic portion sizes listed on most product labels, you could easily be getting two, three, or more grams of these dangerous, artery-clogging fats in one sitting.

Keep in mind the daily amount of trans fats considered safe to consume is ZERO.

Don't Smoke, Just Don't

This edict should go without saying. However, since the Centers for Disease Control and Prevention estimates that approximately 16.5 percent of American women still smoke, some folks still haven't gotten the memo. Smoking doesn't only cause lung cancer, emphysema, and other horrible diseases; ample evidence links the smoking habit to breast cancer, too.

A recent study that analyzed data from over 73,000 women showed that new cases of invasive breast cancer were 24 percent higher in women who currently smoked and 13 percent higher in former smokers than for non-smokers. The statistics are worse for women who began smoking at an early age. Women who started smoking before their first menstrual cycle were 61 percent more likely to develop breast cancer than those who didn't. Those who started after their first cycle but 11 or more years before the birth of their first child were 45 percent more likely to develop the disease.[62]

Of particular interest in this study was that the increased risk for smokers versus non-smokers only occurred in women who also drank alcohol. No increase in risk was noted in women who never drank. Regardless, don't smoke!

So the next time you go out for a glass of wine or a cocktail, skip the cigarette.

30 Dump (Most) Dairy

If you're familiar with The Vail Diet website, you know it's not about dogma or extremes. That said, one food category you'd be best to reduce or even eliminate from your diet is dairy.

In the book *The China Study*, Dr. T. Colin Campbell highlighted the link between animal protein and cancer. Much of his compelling research focused on casein, a protein found in milk. Both laboratory and epidemiological (population) studies indicated a strong link between casein and many types of cancer. Dr. Campbell even called casein "the most relevant cancer promoter ever discovered."

Other studies have also linked consuming high-fat dairy products to breast cancer. Dairy products in general have been linked to both prostate and ovarian cancer. After all, prostate, ovarian, and the majority of breast cancers are hormone driven and dairy products—even organic ones—contain growth hormones.

However, many experts advocating a high-protein diet have criticized Dr. Campbell's methods and conclusions. William Davis, MD, and author of the best-selling book *Wheat Belly*, has pointed to the work of Denise Minger. This young self-taught nutrition writer analyzed Dr. Campbell's data with a fine-toothed comb and concluded he misrepresented many of his findings.[63] Since that came out, many in the health field have questioned her methods and tried to tie her to pro-beef organizations.

Controversy never ends.

What's my advice on dairy? Overall, humans are probably not ideally suited to drink milk throughout life. In fact, we lose more than 90 percent of our lactase (the enzyme necessary to digest dairy) by age five. According to the National Institutes of Health, about 65 percent of the world's population is actually lactose intolerant. While about 90 percent of East Asians are lactose intolerant, this afflicts only about 5 percent of Northern Europeans.[64]

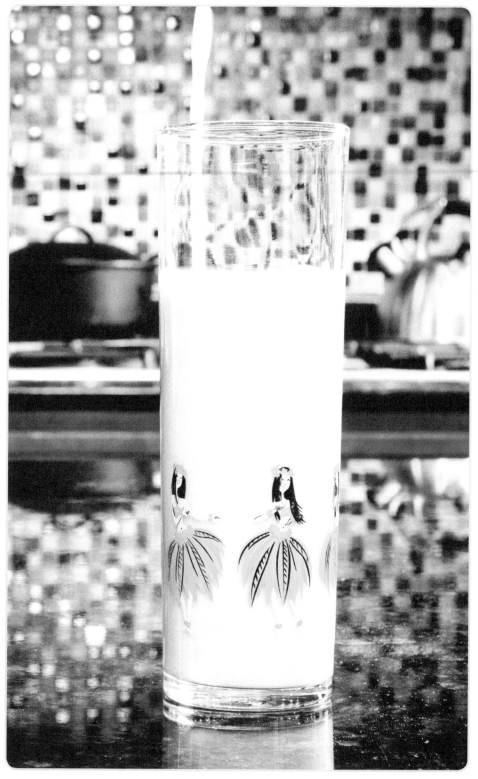

One thing that's known for sure—the massive amounts of cheese and cream sauces served in many restaurant meals lead to chronic disease and should be avoided.

If you choose to eat dairy, do so in moderation and make sure it's high quality.

Lift Safely

Tips for Eating Dairy

If you can't forgo dairy in your diet, follow these recommendations to ensure you're eating it in the healthiest way possible:

- ❀ Ignore government recommendations regarding number of servings a day; these are based on politics, not health. And the numbers are too high for optimal health.

- ❀ No, your bones will not disintegrate without a diet full of dairy. Countries with the highest dairy consumption have the highest rates of hip fractures and vice versa. Instead, get your calcium from leafy green vegetables—like the cows do.

- ❀ Eat yogurt. As mentioned, the beneficial bacteria in yogurt and other fermented foods are crucial to good gut health. In addition, the fermentation process makes yogurt easier to digest than other milk products. However, avoid sweetened yogurts full of artificial flavors, colors, and other chemicals; some of them have as much sugar as a soda. Instead, buy plain organic yogurt and add your own fruit and sweeteners. You will never add as much sweetener as the food companies do.

- ❀ Buy organic. All dairy products contain growth hormones. Remember, the whole point of milk is to make a calf grow in excess of 1,000 pounds in a few short months. Because growth hormones may fuel cancer, why add to that by consuming dairy with added growth hormones? At the very least, look for "no rBGH" (recombinant bovine growth hormone) dairy products.

- ❀ When you buy organic, you avoid taking in antibiotics through the milk. More than 80 percent of the antibiotics produced in the United States go into our food supply. This likely contributes to the growth of antibiotic-resistant superbugs.

Dairy Allergy or Lactose Intolerance?

Dairy allergies and lactose intolerance are terms often erroneously used interchangeably. To set the record straight, they are *not* the same thing.

A dairy allergy results from a malfunctioning immune system. In an allergic reaction, the immune system identifies milk proteins (either casein or whey) as harmful and releases antibodies into your bloodstream. These antibodies release histamine, which causes allergy symptoms similar to that caused by a cold. Dairy allergies can also cause a host of gastrointestinal issues and, in some cases, anaphylaxis—a life-threating reaction that leaves one unable to breathe.

Lactose intolerance is caused by insufficient amounts of lactase, the enzyme necessary to digest lactose, a naturally occurring sugar in milk. Typical symptoms of lactose intolerance may include bloating, gas, and diarrhea.

If you chronically experience any of these symptoms, consider giving up dairy for a few weeks to see how you feel. If your symptoms subside, then it may not be wise to include dairy in your diet.

31 Forget Folic Acid

What is folic acid, and why is it sometimes called folate? Folic acid is the synthetic version of folate used in supplements and fortified foods. Folate, on the other hand, is another word for a water-soluble vitamin known as B9, which occurs naturally in food. This important nutrient protects your DNA from damage, such as drinking alcohol can cause.

Folate is also *crucial* to the proper development of babies in the womb, preventing neural tube defects (NTDs) such as spina bifida. For this reason, food fortification with folic acid was made mandatory in the U.S. in 1998.

The bad news is, high intakes of folic acid have been shown to increase the incidence of cancers of the colon, prostate, and breast. According to one study, women who supplement with folic acid increase their breast cancer risk by 20 to 30 percent.[65] The news for prostate cancer was even worse; one study noted a 163 percent increase in the disease for men taking folic acid.[66]

Folate is not only meant for preventing birth defects. It's still an important vitamin for men and offers many benefits.

How can you ensure adequate levels of folate in your blood? Don't take supplements or eat foods fortified with folic acid. Rather, eat folate-rich foods that include spinach, romaine lettuce, endive, mustard and collard greens, bok choy, arugula, asparagus, broccoli, and many other green vegetables. Tomatoes, beans, lentils, and beef and chicken livers are also good sources of folate.

Most adults can get all the folate they need through diet alone.

Unmarked Obstacles

Folate and Pregnancy

If you're planning to become pregnant, adequate amounts of folate are crucial to a healthy pregnancy. Because birth defects occur in the first few weeks of pregnancy, you need to be concerned about folate as soon as you decide to become pregnant. By the time a woman confirms her pregnancy, it may be too late.

Sadly, many American women do not eat enough folate-rich foods. If that's you, speak to a natural medicine practitioner for guidance ideally *before* becoming pregnant. Your practitioner can help you with your diet and may recommend certain supplements containing a biologically active form of folate rather than synthetic folic acid.

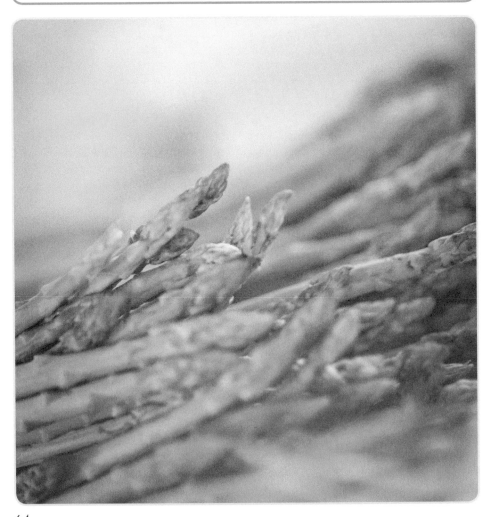

"Heck No" to Added Hormones

Exposure to too much estrogen is linked to breast cancer. In fact, women who began menstruation at age 15 have two-thirds the risk of pre-menopausal breast cancer as those who began at age 11, due to their shorter lifetime exposure to estrogen. With so much estrogen we're naturally exposed to, why add to that problem by eating foods with added growth hormones?

In 1993, the FDA approved Monsanto's genetically modified recombinant bovine growth hormone (rBGH), also known as recombinant bovine somatotrophin (rBST). To increase milk production, this hormone is injected into dairy cows and can be found in all types of dairy products including milk, cheese, ice cream, and yogurt.

Injecting cows with these hormones causes an increase in insulin-like growth factor (IGF-1), which already occurs naturally in both animals and humans. While this substance is important during childhood growth, excessive amounts can promote abnormal cell growth in an adult *and* have been linked to increased cancer risk.

Specifically, a global body of evidence indicates that higher IGF-1 levels in the blood increase the risk of estrogen receptor positive breast cancer.[67]

On top of that, most cattle in the U.S. are given extra estrogen to make them fatter. Therefore, eating any meat or dairy can raise your IGF-1 levels, but *eating meat or milk from an animal treated with rBGH, rBST, or estrogen is even worse.*

If you must ingest beef or drink cow's milk, do so in moderation and buy organic. Remember, labeling laws for organic certification don't allow the animal to be treated with growth hormones. The USDA does not allow chickens, turkeys, or hogs in the U.S. to be treated with added hormones; however, because you're still ingesting their *natural* hormones, be sure you eat moderate amounts of their meat.

 ## Pass on Processed Meats

Processed meats include deli/luncheon meats, ham, bacon, bologna, salami, hot dogs, and others. Why avoid them? Because they contain preservatives called sodium nitrate and sodium nitrite, which manufacturers use to inhibit the growth of harmful bacteria and preserve their pink or red color.

Nitrates and nitrites sometimes turn into harmless substances in the gut. However, they can also turn into molecules called nitrosamines, which have been shown to cause cancer in animals. The World Cancer Research fund offers convincing evidence that processed (and red) meats cause colorectal cancer.[68]

In addition, a recent study of almost 450,000 people found significant associations with processed meat intake and cancer, cardiovascular diseases, and "other causes of death."[69]

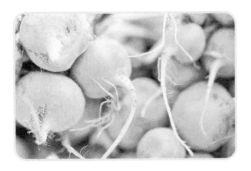
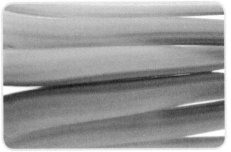

Nitrates and nitrites are also found in certain vegetables, including spinach, radishes, celery, lettuce, beets, and root vegetables. So the association between nitrates/nitrites and cancer may be related more to how they're delivered—in hot dogs vs. spinach. In other words, an ingredient other than nitrates or nitrites in processed meats may be the cancer-causing culprit.

My opinion, shared by many nutritional experts, is to avoid eating processed meats altogether. If you absolutely must eat them, do so sparingly and buy organic brands that don't have added hormones, antibiotics, nitrates, or nitrites.

Lift Safely
Vitamin C vs. Nitrosamines

When my sister and I were kids and my mom occasionally fed us hot dogs (typically natural brands made with turkey), she always gave us a vitamin C with our meal. Today, I understand why. Vitamin C can promote the formation of nitric oxide, which blocks the formation of nitrosamines in the gut. So when you do eat processed meat, take a vitamin C on the side.

Thanks for the tip, Mom!

 ## Say NO to GMOs!

GMOs are animals and plants that have been genetically engineered by scientists to exhibit particular traits. These traits can include speeded-up growing cycles and/or the ability to withstand certain herbicides and pesticides.

Beware: Salmon that grows at twice the normal rate due to fancy genetic engineering that keeps their production of growth hormones permanently "on" will likely hit grocery stores in the near future.

These days, quite a debate is raging regarding the safety of genetically modified organisms or GMOs. The biotech industry claims GMOs are safe, yet more than 60 nations in the world have significantly restricted or banned their production and sale.[70]

According to Dr. Thierry Vrain, a former biotech researcher and GMO supporter, most research sponsored by the biotech industry shows the technology is safe, while most research performed by foreign agencies and universities shows serious problems with the technology.[71]

Funny how that works.

One 2012 study conducted in France showed two to three times more rats fed GM corn died than of those that did not receive the corn, and they died more rapidly. In addition, the GM-corn-fed rats developed large mammary tumors more often and earlier than the control population in most cases. Plus they exhibited liver damage and digestive problems.[72] *Note:* This study has been widely questioned by many scientists due to insufficient sample sizes and the propensity of the type of rats used to develop tumors.

Both sides see this 2012 French study as the end of the story. To some, it proves that GMOs are completely unsafe and to others, the real or perceived lack of discipline in this study renders its findings meaningless. At the very least, it should indicate that far more research needs to be done to prove the safety of GM foods before they are forced on consumers—in many cases, against our will and with no warning label.

Until more is known, it seems unwise to blindly follow the side that profits from this genetic engineering technology.

My advice? Avoid genetically modified foods, period. The best choice is to buy whole foods labeled "certified organic" so you can be 100 percent sure you're not consuming GMOs. *Note:* Current organic regulations in the U.S. prohibit the use of GMOs.

Another way to identify non-GMO food is to look for this "Non-GMO Project" label:

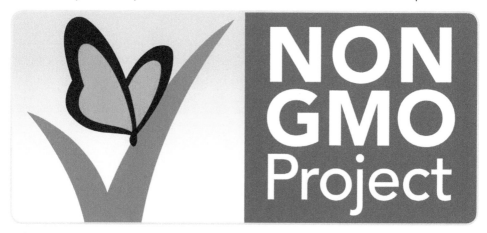

What position on consumer safety does Monsanto, the world's largest producer of GMO seeds, take? In 1998, the company's director of corporate communications had this to say to the *New York Times Magazine*: "Monsanto should not have to vouchsafe the safety of biotech food. Our interest is in selling as much of it as possible. Assuring its safety is the U.S. Food and Drug Administration's job."[73]

'Nuff said.

Unmarked Obstacles

Most Common GMO/GE Foods

Listed here are the most frequently genetically modified/engineered foods:

- ✿ Corn
- ✿ Soybeans
- ✿ Tomatoes
- ✿ Papaya
- ✿ Canola oil (also called rapeseed)
- ✿ Milk (when it contains the genetically modified recombinant bovine growth hormone—rBGH or recombinant bovine somatotrophin—rBST)
- ✿ Aspartame
- ✿ Beet sugar
- ✿ Zucchini and yellow squash
- ✿ Rice

With corn and/or some form of soy appearing in almost every processed food, it means more than 80 percent of the processed food supply in the U.S. contains GMO ingredients. That's why it's critical to diligently stick with foods labeled "organic" and avoid GMOs. For more information check out the EWG's Shoppers Guide to Avoiding GE Foods at www.ewg.org/research/shoppers-guide-to-avoiding-ge-food.

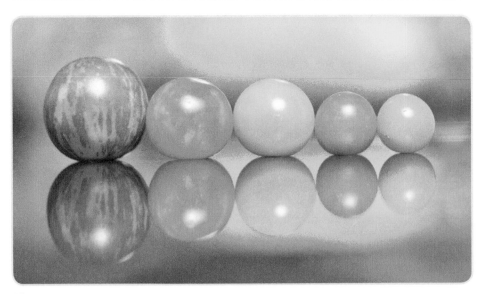

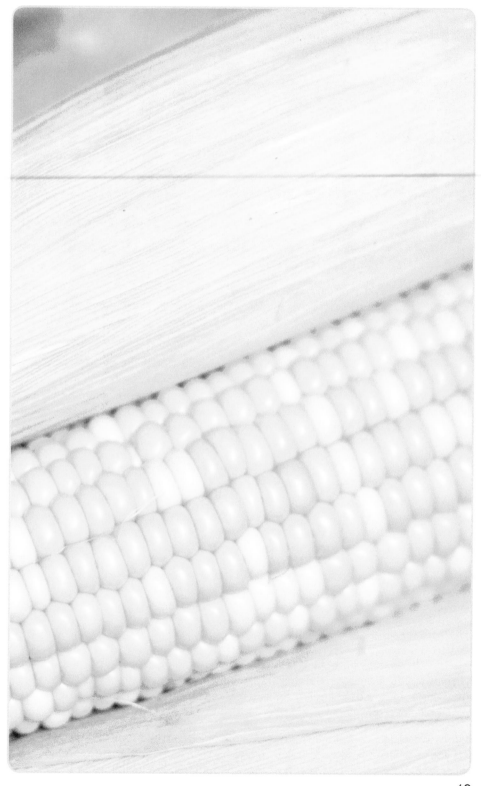

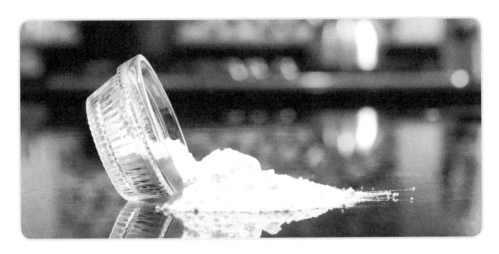

35 Shun the White Stuff

By white stuff, I'm talking white flour and refined sugar, white or not. To your body's digestive system, sugar and white flour are essentially the same. During digestion, flour quickly converts to sugar and puts stress on the pancreas, which is then required to release large amounts of insulin for digestion.

Did you know that sugar consumption is on the rise? In 1830, the average American ate approximately 12 pounds of sugar each year; by 1930, that figure rose to 109 pounds.[74] Nowadays, Americans eat and drink an average of more than 150 pounds of sugar each year. In addition, overconsumption of processed cookies and crackers, cakes, white bread, and pasta leads to Americans eating a steady stream of white flour, too.

Population and laboratory studies have shown a link between cancer and insulin resistance, a condition caused by the consumption of excessive sugar and/or white flour.[75] Another study showed significant risks for breast and colorectal cancer as the intake of starchy refined cereals increased.[76] In addition to cancer, eating too much white stuff causes inflammation in the body. Inflammation, a primary cause of type-2 diabetes, eventually damages one's heart.

When it comes to sugar, the poison is in the dose. Because our bodies need glucose, we can handle *some* sugar. However, they're simply not designed to handle the enormous amounts we are eating today. Combine that with a sedentary lifestyle and we have a society in which chronic diseases run rampant.

To cut sugar out of your diet, stop drinking sugary beverages—now! Soda, fruit juices, bottled teas, lemonade, vitamin-enhanced beverages—all the same to your pancreas. But don't replace them with artificially sweetened beverages, which are just as unhealthy for different reasons. (See Tip 27 to learn more about artificial sweeteners.)

Start by watering down or cutting back on the number of sugary drinks you consume until you've whittled it down to none. Turn to healthy substitutes instead, such as homemade green juice, or water flavored with real fruit like lemon, lime, straw berry, watermelon, or cucumber. The possibilities are endless. Unsweetened iced herbal tea is also a good option.

To sweeten home-baked goods, use raw organic honey, organic palm sugar, or pure maple syrup—all better choices than highly processed, genetically modified table sugar. *Note:* Even natural sweeteners should be eaten in extreme moderation. The maximum amount recommended is 6 teaspoons daily for women and 9 teaspoons for men.

To reduce white flour in your diet, start by eliminating processed cookies, crackers, cakes, and so on. Change your bread to whole grain, sprouted wheat, or sourdough. (Sourdough bread doesn't spike your blood sugar as much as others; it's easier to digest and even contains good gut bacteria.) Avoid "wheat" bread made with highly processed flour and caramel coloring. Buy pasta made with Jerusalem artichoke flour rather than regular pasta. It tastes the same, but it doesn't cause the same blood sugar spike.

Go easy consuming the white stuff and choose healthier options instead!

Unmarked Obstacles
Beware of Hidden Sugar

Food manufacturers do an amazing job of hiding sugar in our food, using dozens of code words for it in their labeling. Be your own food detective and watch out for hidden sugars masquerading under these and other names:

- ❀ Barley
- ❀ Malt
- ❀ Caramel
- ❀ Concentrate juice
- ❀ Corn sugar
- ❀ Disaccharide
- ❀ High fructose corn syrup
- ❀ Maize syrup
- ❀ Malt syrup
- ❀ Molasses
- ❀ Sorbitol
- ❀ Sucanat
- ❀ Turbinado
- ❀ Just about any word ending in "ose"

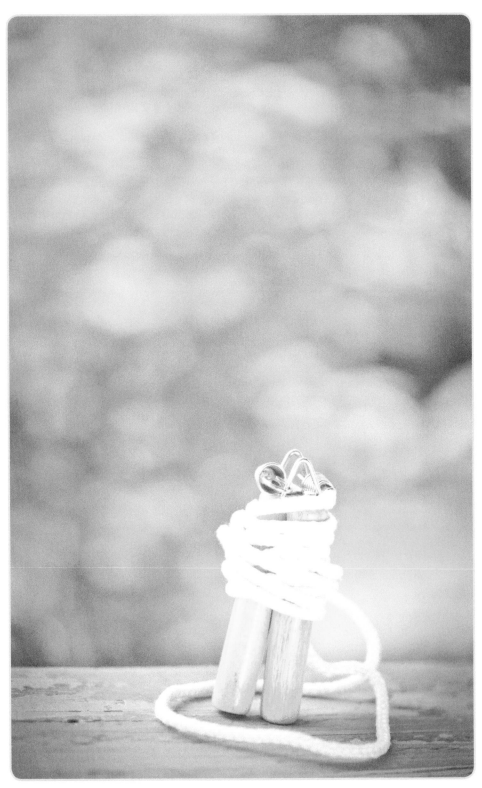

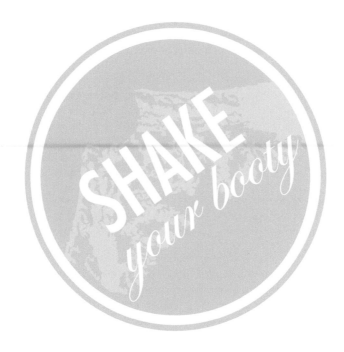

Study after study has shown the importance of physical activity in preventing obesity and heart disease. But did you know it's also strongly linked to preventing cancer? The following five tips will have you shakin' your booty and reducing your risk of cancer in no time.

Circumvent the Chair (and Couch!)

You don't need to hit the gym to benefit from physical activity, but you do need to get out of the chair and off the couch! The past few years have seen an onslaught of press about the dangers of sitting. *And the news ain't good.* In April 2012, the *New York Times* called the disastrous consequences of sitting "swift, pervasive and punishing."[77]

We've known since the early 1950s that sitting is terrible for one's health. Back then, a study of London bus conductors and drivers showed that the conductors were leaner and died of heart disease at half the rate as the drivers. The reason? As ticket collectors, the conductors regularly walked through the bus and up and down the stairs. The drivers, however, stayed behind the wheel for most of the day.[78]

More recently, a study linked nearly 90,000 new cancer cases a year to lack of physical activity or prolonged periods of sitting, including 49,000 cases of breast cancer.[79] In addition, a 2012 meta-analysis of 18 studies that included close to 800,000 participants showed that sitting for prolonged periods increased the risk of diabetes (112 percent increase), cardiovascular events (147 percent increase), death from cardiovascular events (90 percent increase), and death from all causes (49 percent increase).[80]

Why is sitting so dangerous? Because our bodies were designed for walking and movement, not sitting on our behinds for hours on end. For thousands of years, exercise occurred naturally. However, today, people spend half of their waking hours sitting. And unfortunately, exercising doesn't necessarily let you off the hook. An eight-year study of 250,000 American adults showed that exercise had only a small effect on the risk of death for those who were otherwise sedentary.[77]

How can you mitigate the negative effects of prolonged inactivity? The key is to increase activity level *throughout the day*, not only in one spurt at the beginning or end. Even a two-minute walk every 20 minutes can improve your glucose metabolism.

Think of an hour at work as a therapist would-that is, as a 50-minute hour. Then spend five to ten minutes an hour moving around. Your body will thank you and a smart employer will endorse the practice. Health care savings and increased productivity should more than compensate for those lost minutes of work.

37) Pump Some Iron

Getting aerobic exercise such as walking isn't the only way to improve your fitness level. You can reduce your insulin and hormone levels (along with your chances of developing breast cancer) by lifting weights or doing other forms of weight-bearing exercise. In addition, weight training can help survivors regain their strength and muscle tone during and after chemotherapy and/or radiation treatments, while increasing their energy.

Unfortunately, in the past, breast cancer survivors were instructed to not lift anything heavier than five pounds due to the perceived risk of lymphedema (buildup of lymph fluids that can cause mild to severe arm swelling). However, according to a 2006 study of 45 breast cancer survivors, weight training did *not* increase the risk for or exacerbate symptoms of lymphedema.[81]

Not all weight training needs to take place in a gym. Your own body weight works perfectly for building and toning muscle. Start with good old-fashioned calisthenics like rope jumping, push-ups, sit-ups, squats, and burpees. Invest in a set of dumbbells and, several times a week, do two to three sets of six to eight exercises that work several major muscle groups.

Performing a strategic combination of cardio and strength training is one of the most effective ways to keep in shape.

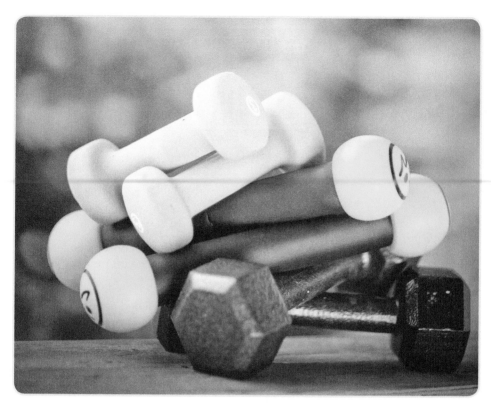

38 Walk 'Til You Drop

Taking frequent walks is one of the best ways to reduce your risk of developing breast cancer. Free and easy, walking can either be a social activity or blissfully solitary.

A study conducted by the American Cancer Society tracked almost 74,000 post-menopausal women for 17 years. The researchers found that those who walked seven hours or more each week had a 14 percent lower risk of developing breast cancer than those who walked three hours or less. In addition, women who exercised vigorously for one hour a day had a 25 percent lower risk of developing the disease. (This lower risk was true for both estrogen receptor positive and estrogen receptor negative breast cancers.) Even more encouraging—the prevention benefits applied to women of all weight levels.[82]

And walking isn't only useful for preventing cancer. It also enhances the quality of life and energy levels in patients and survivors, while greatly improving a person's mood. Experts aren't sure how or why walking helps prevent breast cancer, but they believe it may be due to better regulated hormone levels.

Commit to walking two or more miles several days a week. While any walking speed is better for you than sitting, it's best to walk at a moderate pace of three to four miles an hour to achieve maximum benefits.

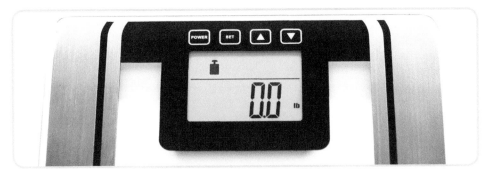

39 Watch Your Weight

Prevent breast cancer by maintaining a healthy body weight. Not only are overweight women more likely to develop breast cancer than lean women, but they're also more likely to have a recurrence of the disease—or die from it.

This conclusion is backed by one study in particular that included nearly 7,000 women. It showed that obese (20 percent or more over ideal body weight) women have a 30 percent greater chance of disease recurrence and are 69 percent more likely to die from breast cancer or other causes than women of normal weight. Women who were overweight but not obese also showed an increased chance of recurrence or death.[83]

This negative effect of weight on breast cancer recurrence and death occurred to the greatest extent in women with estrogen receptor positive breast cancers. (Weight was not as strongly linked to estrogen receptor negative breast cancers.) The risk also appears to apply primarily to women after menopause. That's when the ovaries no longer produce estrogen; therefore, any estrogen in the body is primarily produced by fat tissues.

How and why does weight affect your chances of developing breast cancer? One possible reason for this increased risk is that overweight women produce more estrogen than women of normal weight, and estrogen fuels estrogen receptor positive breast cancer. Overweight people also produce more insulin, which can stimulate the growth of breast cancer cells.

So, exactly what is a healthy weight? Overall, a healthy body mass index (BMI) for women is from 18.5 to 24.9, with the healthiest range being from 22.0 to 23.5.[84] However, keep in mind that BMI doesn't perfectly measure how healthy your weight is. Specifically, it doesn't measure the level of fat in your body, which is one of the most important indicators of health.

That said, your BMI can be a useful tool to give you a general idea of where you stack up health wise.

Don't despair! You can reap many benefits from decreasing your body weight, even a small amount. Research shows that losing just 5 percent of your body weight can cut your risk of estrogen positive breast cancer by 22 percent.[85]

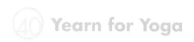 Yearn for Yoga

Why is yoga good for you? First, it can help prevent breast cancer. Doing yoga can keep you lean and fit, which reduces the production of estrogen and insulin—both factors in breast cancer and other types of cancer. Yoga also boosts t-cells, which are crucial cells in your body's immune response.

But that's not all of yoga's known benefits. It:

- Improves circulation,

- Relaxes you and reduces your stress,

- Strengthens your immune system by stimulating lymph flow,

- Regulates your endocrine system by increasing circulation during inversion poses, and

- Puts you in a healthier and more holistic mindset. (Most folks don't leave yoga class and race out for a cigarette or fast food burger.)

Recent studies have also shown that yoga affects the quality of life for breast cancer survivors by improving sleep, reducing fatigue, and increasing physical vitality.[86] Certain yogic breathing exercises can even help control nausea.

What type of yoga works best? With many different types of yoga available—from less physically demanding restorative kinds to rigorous yoga done in a room heated to over 100 degrees—the best one is whichever you enjoy most. And that's most likely the one you'll stick with!

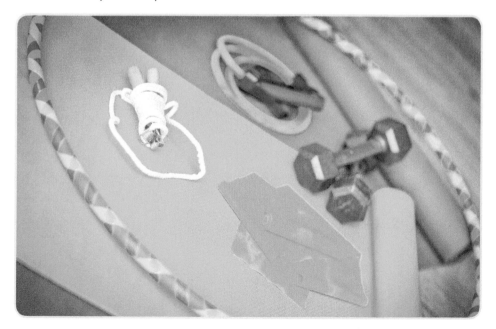

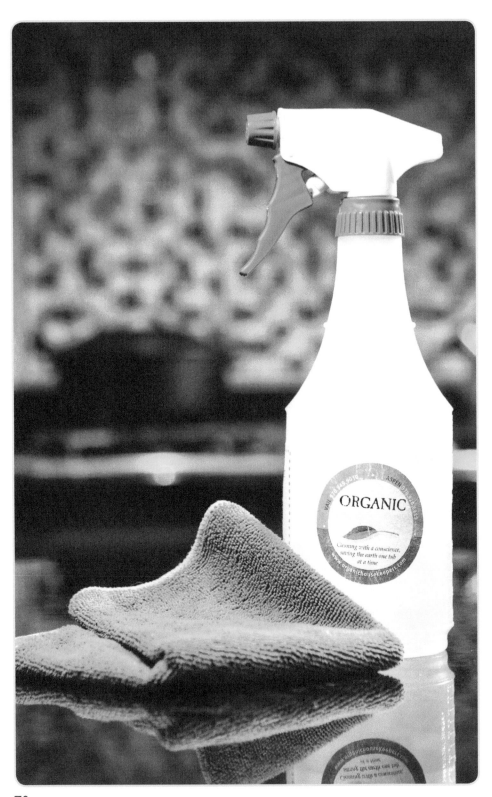

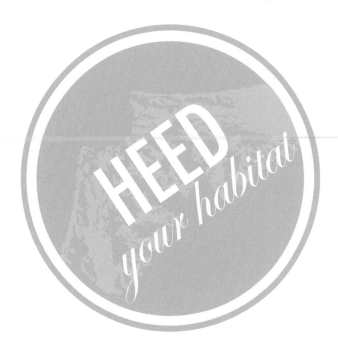

Our environment is filled with potentially dangerous chemicals. Thousands of them can be found in beauty, personal care, and cleaning products. Most of them have never been tested for safety or faced regulatory scrutiny. In addition, the water supply in most communities contains hundreds of potentially dangerous chemicals, the majority of which are also unregulated.

Here are five steps you can take to protect yourself from some of the worst offenders:

(41) Abolish Aluminum

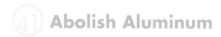 Aluminum, an element on the periodic table, is the second most commonly used metal today. While it's extremely useful in the transportation and other industries, does it belong in your antiperspirant or deodorant? This point is under debate, with no conclusive research linking the use of underarm antiperspirants and deodorants to breast cancer. Yet, some evidence does exist.

In theory, the potential dangers of aluminum in antiperspirant involve the skin absorbing it and depositing it in breast tissue, thus causing changes in breast cells' estrogen receptors. And because estrogen can fuel breast cancer cells, some scientists believe using these products may lead to developing the disease.

Studies show conflicting results. For instance, a 2002 study that compared 813 women with breast cancer to 793 without the disease did not show increased risks for breast cancer in women who use underarm antiperspirants or deodorants, or who shave under their arms. Yet a 2003 study that included 437 breast cancer survivors found that the age of diagnosis was significantly earlier for women who shaved their underarms frequently and used antiperspirant or deodorant. In addition, the age of diagnosis was even earlier for women who began these habits before the age of 16.[87]

So what should you do? First, consider switching from antiperspirant to deodorant, since aluminum is *usually* only found in antiperspirant and a little sweat is good for you. Sweating is one the body's natural detoxification processes.

Whichever you choose, deodorant or antiperspirant, check the label for the words aluminum or alum. (While alum is safer than aluminum, it's not completely aluminum free.) Also check for plenty of other nasty chemicals in your deodorant, such as parabens and toxic fragrances.

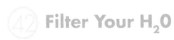 Filter Your H$_2$O

Some government officials love to tout the cleanliness of their cities' drinking water, even comparing it to champagne. In fact, tap water can be more like a toxic soup of hundreds of potentially dangerous chemicals.

Between 2004 and 2009, the Environmental Working Group (EWG) analyzed the results of almost 20 million tests of drinking water performed by water suppliers. It found hundreds of contaminants and, in many cases, the chemicals exceeded existing safety limits.[88]

In addition, two-thirds of the 315 chemicals identified by the EWG are unregulated. *That means no limit exists on how many or how much of these chemicals can end up in your drinking water.* While most water suppliers keep the amount of these contaminants below government limits, far too many chemicals have no stated government limits at all.

Toxic substances found in water supplies include the following:

❀ Agricultural chemicals such as fertilizers and pesticides,

❀ Industrial chemicals such as those used in plastics,

❀ Byproducts from water disinfecting processes, and

❀ Arsenic, chloroform, and perchlorate (i.e., rocket fuel).

Many of these chemicals (some known to be highly carcinogenic) can damage the thyroid, liver, kidneys, nervous system, and immune system. They're also capable of causing birth defects and miscarriages.

Filtering the drinking water in your home is crucial—but that's not enough. It's important to filter the water throughout your home, including your bathroom. Chlorine, a toxic chemical used as a disinfectant by almost every water supplier in the U.S., can enter your body through your pores when you shower or bathe. In addition, the heat from the water can cause chlorine gas to form. When inhaled, the gas goes straight into your bloodstream.

So for optimum health, filter all of the water in your home.

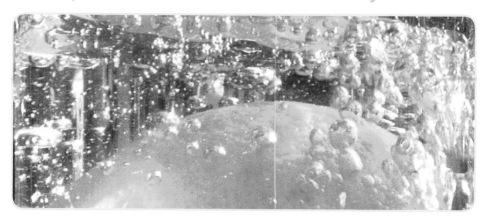

Lift Safely

There's WHAT in My Water?

As if the chemicals mentioned aren't bad enough, tap water also typically contains a myriad of pharmaceutical drugs. Please do the environment a favor: Do *not* flush expired or unneeded over-the-counter drugs down the toilet. Save them (well out of reach of children) in an empty carton or container and bring them to your city or town for proper disposal.

For information on your local water supply, additional tips for safer water, and the best filter for your needs, visit the EWG's National Drinking Water Database at www.ewg.org/tap-water.

 Green Your Cleaning Products

Buyer beware. If the American public understood that very few of the chemicals used in modern cleaning products have ever been tested for safety, far fewer people would endorse that "clean" smell of a home bathed in toxic chemicals.

Silent Spring Institute is an organization formed in 1994 to investigate elevated breast cancer rates on Cape Cod. Its research, based on phone interviews with 1,500 women, showed that women who report using the most cleaning products had double the rate of breast cancer as those who reported using the least. Air fresheners, products to control mold and mildew, and insect repellents were the products most strongly linked to breast cancer.[89] *Note:* Some medical experts as well as the manufacturers of cleaning products expressed criticism of this study.

Frankly, not a lot of data exists on cleaning products and breast cancer. There's simply no financial incentive for any company or organization to spend large amounts of money on studies like this. However, we do know these products are *loaded with* toxic chemicals. Many of them have been labeled human carcinogens, others are called endocrine disruptors, and some remain in fat tissues for years. Still others include toxic heavy metals linked to a myriad of diseases.

Ditch toxic cleaning products, especially if you have children. Being around chemical overload is more dangerous to their tiny bodies than to adults' bodies. So purchase "green" cleaning products, but also be beware of "greenwashing." It's a term describing companies that give lip service to going green while sneaking nasty chemicals into their products under less-recognizable names.

Better yet, make your own cleaning products. Not only will they be safe and effective, you'll know *exactly* what's in them.

Unmarked Obstacles

What's in Your Cleaning Products?

The following are just a fraction of the hundreds of chemicals used in cleaning products, with their potential effects on your body:

- ❀ Ammonia – can irritate eyes and lungs and cause headaches.

- ❀ Formaldehyde – used as a preservative in many products; possible human carcinogen and irritant of eyes, throat, lungs, and skin.

- ❀ Naphthalene – in mothballs, possible human carcinogen that can damage the eyes, blood cells, liver, kidneys, skin, and central nervous system.

- ❀ Nitrobenzene – in furniture and floor polishes; can cause shallow breathing and death if ingested.

- ❀ Hydrochloric acid – in toilet bowl cleaners, can burn the skin and stomach if ingested, and can cause blindness if splashed into the eyes.

- ❀ Fragrances. While this word conjures up images of wildflowers in a field, this couldn't be further from the truth. One fragrance can be made up of hundreds of dangerous chemicals, and you'll never know what they are because the list of ingredients in a fragrance is protected by intellectual property laws.

To find out how safe your favorite cleaners are, check out the EWG's Guide to Healthy Cleaning at www.ewg.org/guides/cleaners.

Do-It-Yourself Cleaning Products

Here are a few green-cleaning product ingredients you may already have in your home:

❀ White vinegar – an effective disinfectant for some pathogens but not all. Will not kill some types of salmonella so use something stronger for kitchen counters. White vinegar diluted in water is ideal for cleaning mirrors and hardwood floors.

❀ Vodka – my personal favorite. Using a mixture of one-part vodka to four parts water makes an effective surface cleaner. It works great to clean countertops and appliances (and who cares if a little gets on your food).

❀ Hydrogen peroxide – an effective sanitizer. Use a 3% solution on kitchen and bathroom countertops as well as disinfect fruits and vegetables and brighten your whites in the laundry.

❀ Club soda – removes some stains from carpets if applied immediately after a spill.

❀ Baking soda – good for removing grime from porcelain, tile, kitchen counters, and the inside of an oven. It can also be used with boiling water to unclog a drain.

❀ Essential oils – not only do these add a lovely smell to your do-it-yourself cleaning products, but certain oils may also be antibacterial, antifungal, or antiseptic.

❀ Castile soap – good old-fashioned soap and water. Dr. Bronner's is a fantastic "green" option.

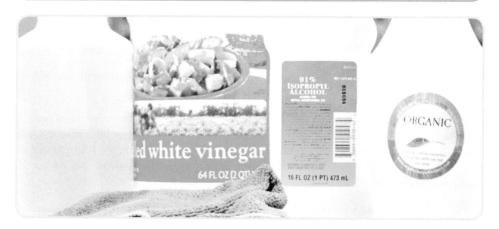

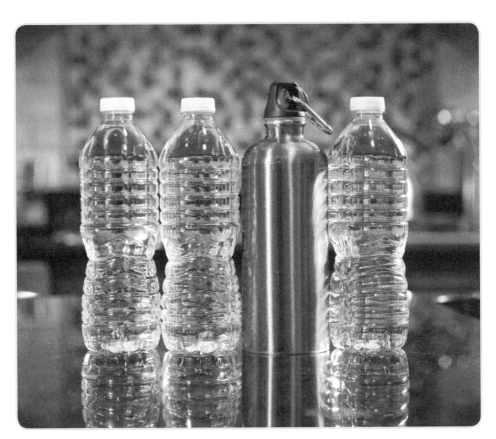

 Pitch the Plastic

Plastic is everywhere. We eat it, drink it, sit on it, wear it, touch it, and spread it all over our bodies. While versatile, inexpensive plastic has revolutionized our world, it's come at a cost to both the environment and our health. Plastic contains many chemicals, two of the most widely used and dangerous being bisphenol-A (commonly called BPA) and phthalates.

BPA is a known endocrine disruptor, which means it alters the normal functioning of our hormones. It mimics estrogen and is believed to stimulate the growth of breast cancer and other reproductive system cancers. BPA has also been linked to early puberty, obesity, hyperactivity, type 2 diabetes, heart disease, fertility issues, and miscarriage. Sadly, this chemical is found everywhere, with approximately six billion pounds of BPA produced globally each year.[90]

Phthalates, another common chemical in plastic, have been shown to interfere with testosterone and other male hormones, and can affect normal sexual development. Like BPA, phthalates are also linked to fertility issues and miscarriage. And phthalates aren't only found in plastic; they're also commonly used in beauty and personal care products in the U.S.

Avoid these chemicals by minimally using plastics in your home.

Discovery Center

Tips for Safer Plastic Use

Here are a few suggestions for decreased and safer use of plastics:

✿ Don't drink water bottled in plastic.

✿ Don't reuse one-use plastic water bottles.

✿ When you're on the go, drink filtered water out of a reusable stainless steel or glass bottle, or use a BPA-free plastic filter bottle.

✿ Get a stainless steel sippy cup for your child and carefully select plastic toys, teething rings, and anything else that may end up in their mouth. These chemicals have a much greater effect on their tiny bodies than adult bodies.

✿ Don't let plastic containers get too hot or cold. Excessive heat or cold may cause the plastic to break down and leach chemicals into your water or food. Don't leave plastic water bottles in your car; don't microwave in plastic (no matter what the packaging says); don't freeze food in plastic containers.

✿ Don't store leftover food, especially hot food, in plastic containers. Instead, use glass containers such as those made by Pyrex®.

✿ BPA is also commonly found in food can liners, so minimize your use of canned foods or look for cans marked "BPA free." Companies using BPA-free can liners include Eden, Native Forest, Wild Planet, Farmer's Market, and Muir Glen.

✿ BPA is not just found in plastic. A significant percentage of paper receipts in the U.S. contain the chemical. Leave the receipt unless you really need it.

✿ Use safe, environmentally friendly cosmetics, perfumes, personal care and cleaning products, laundry detergent, and dish soap to avoid dangerous phthalates and other chemicals.

✿ Plastic shower curtains are loaded with phthalates and PVCs; buy one that's free of these and other potentially dangerous chemicals.

For more information on the dangers of endocrine disruptors, check out the EWG's Dirty Dozen of Endocrine Disruptors at www.ewg.org/research/dirty-dozen-list-endocrine-disruptors.

Important Note: The EWG is looking out for us when so many corporations are not. Please consider donating to them at Ways to Donate at www.ewg.org/support-our-work/ways-to-donate.

Purge the Parabens (and Other Junk)

Did you know that what you put on your skin ends up in your bloodstream within about 30 seconds? When you consider that most women use 20 or more different products a day, that translates into a boatload of chemicals. Some experts estimate that women absorb almost five pounds of chemicals a year from cosmetics use alone.[91]

Among the worst chemicals—and most prevalent—are parabens. Because they prohibit the growth of bacteria, yeast, and mold, parabens are used as a preservative in personal care products such as lotions, shampoos, conditioners, cosmetics, antiperspirants, deodorants, toothpaste, and many others. They're also used in food and pharmaceutical products. The body absorbs parabens either through the skin or the intestinal tract, depending on whether they are applied to the body or ingested.

Parabens can increase your risk of breast cancer in several ways. First, they act as an endocrine disruptor and mimic estrogen. They also increase expression of genes that cause breast tumor cells to grow. And they've been linked to early puberty, which can also increase the risk of developing breast cancer.

Researchers have found parabens in actual breast tumors. One study that included 40 women being treated for breast cancer found paraben esters in 99 percent of their tumors. In 60 percent of the women, five different paraben esters were found in their tumors.[92] This doesn't necessarily prove the chemical *caused* the tumors, but it's alarming information nonetheless.

Add to parabens tens of thousands of different chemicals used in personal care products today. And virtually none of them are tested for safety.

Due to loopholes in federal law, the FDA cannot require companies to test their ingredients or products for safety before selling them to the public. Yeah, you read that right. Outrageous, isn't it?

Of course, all of the manufacturers claim their products are safe because they only contain "trace amounts" of the chemicals. The problem is, if you use a dozen or more products each day, exactly how "trace" are those amounts in total?

Discovery Center
Make Over Your Makeup Bag

Replacing all your old beauty products at once can be an expensive and daunting task. To ease your mind and your wallet, replace items as you run out instead of all at once. Luckily, loads of great natural brands exist—one of the hottest trends in beauty. You will have a blast experimenting with some of the incredible new products!

For more information on this topic, check out my bible for clean beauty, *No More Dirty Looks* by Siobhan O'Connor and Alexandra Spunt.

How do your favorite products rate for safety? Find out at the EWG's Skin Deep® Cosmetics Database at www.ewg.org/skindeep.

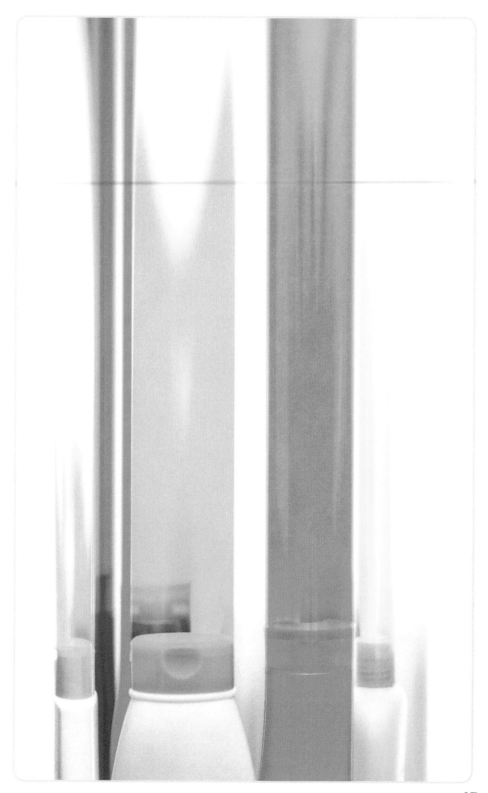

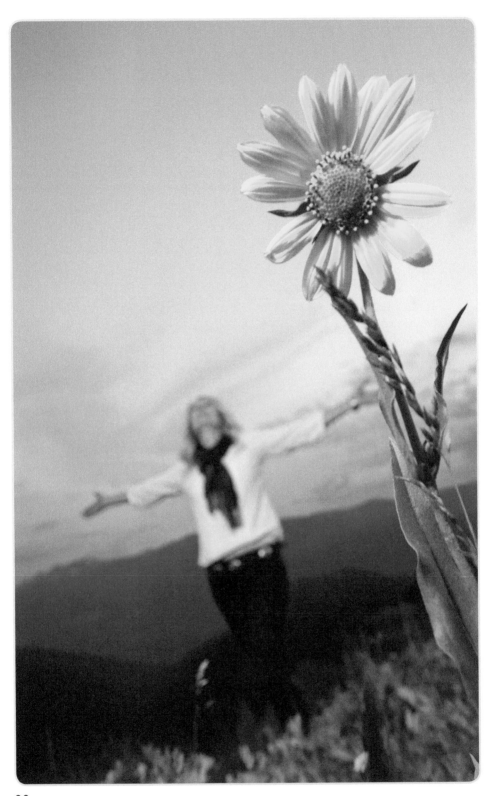

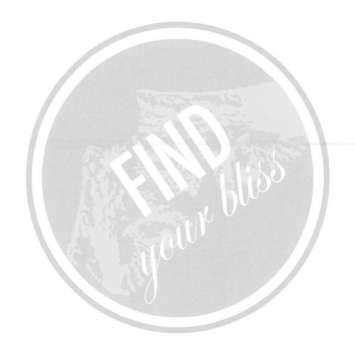

Truly optimal health involves more than what you eat or drink, or how much exercise you get. You can do everything right, but if your mind is like a continuous loop of negative thoughts or you feel stressed out 24/7, you leave yourself open to diseases such as cancer, diabetes, heart disease, depression, and more.

Following these five suggestions will help you relax your mind, reduce your stress, and ultimately, find your bliss.

Don't Stress About Stress

Too much stress can cause a plethora of health problems. Stress and the stress hormone cortisol are addressed in the "Mind Your Mind" section on page 92. But in a nutshell, cortisol has been linked to increased death rates in women with advanced breast cancer.

As you know, stress is difficult to avoid. It's a part of our lives throughout the day, every day. But what if you can change its outcome by adjusting the way you view stress? According to a fascinating TED talk given by Stanford University psychologist Kelly McGonigal, this is possible. (View Kelly McGonigal's TED talk at www.ted.com/talks.)

A study Ms. McGonigal cited found that people who had experienced a lot of stress in the past year had a 43 percent increased risk of dying. However, those who experienced stress but don't believe that stress is harmful to their health had the lowest risk of dying of anyone in the study. It was even lower than those who didn't experience much stress at all.

Ms. McGonigal encouraged listeners to change the way they think about stress, viewing it as your energized body preparing you to meet a particular challenge. Even when the heart is pounding, the blood vessels will stay relaxed when you view the stress response as helpful.

According to Ms. McGonigal's talk, another way to mitigate the potential dangers of stress is to help others. One study tracked about 1,000 adults in the U.S. and found a 30 percent greater chance of dying for every major stressful life experience. However, no increase in stress-related deaths was found in people who had spent time helping others during the past year.

So while stress is unavoidable, its negative health effects are not. Start by helping others. And next time you feel that adrenaline pumping and a stress response coming on, consider it your friend. This one small change in how you view stress may even save your life.

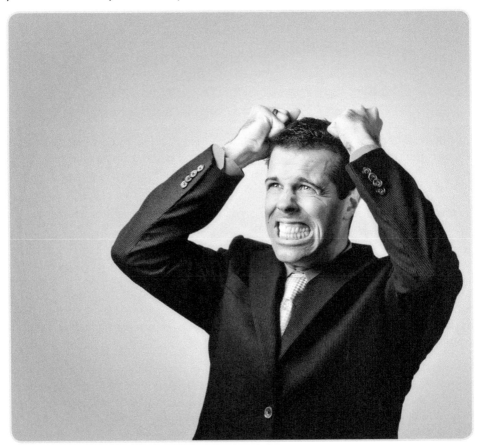

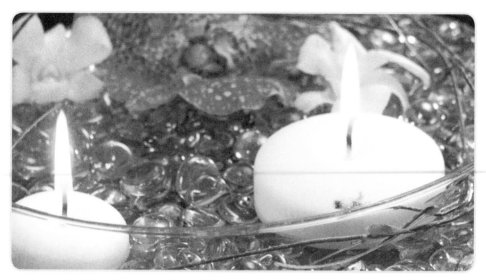

47 Meet Your Masseuse

You've probably heard about the stress-reducing effects of massage therapy. You may even be aware of the positive effects of massage on breast cancer patients, which include less anxiety, less depression, and less anger.[93] These may be psychological, but because of the mind-body connection, they can translate into real physical benefits.

You might also indulge in a massage for its immune-boosting, detoxifying benefits. Massage therapy stimulates the flow of lymph fluid, which allows for the delivery of immune cells throughout the body. (See page 102 for a short explanation of the lymphatic system.) If lymph fluid doesn't flow freely, toxins can accumulate in your body and lead to illness and disease.

Getting massages frequently can be pricey, but I encourage you to treat yourself to one occasionally. Every week or two would be ideal, but do what your lifestyle and budget allow. You can also give an effective massage to yourself or enlist a loved one. I can't say enough about the healing power of touch.

Now for the highly interesting new technique. Recent research has shown that a compressive force (a squeeze) applied to the breasts themselves may guide malignant mammary cells back into a normal growth pattern. Plus, it indicated that although the genetic mutation causing the malignancy remained, the cells stopped growing even after the compression had been removed.[94] That said, it's too soon to say whether this will prevent breast cancer, and it should not be considered a treatment for the disease.

For someone constantly on the lookout for breast cancer prevention tips, this one came as a total surprise to me. Asking your local masseuse to do this type of massage may get you booted from the spa, but it may be worth doing in the privacy of your own home. Experiment!

It's hard to be truly healthy if your mind hangs out in a negative place. In your quest for good health, your extremely powerful mind can either be your ally or your foe.

Unfortunately, for many, the mind can behave like an undisciplined child. This can lead to constant stress and chaos in daily living. *But it doesn't have to be that way.* You can quiet and focus your mind—and achieve an inner calm—through a regular meditation practice.

Little research is available on the direct effects of meditation in preventing breast cancer. However, meditation does reduce stress and thus the release of the stress hormone, cortisol. This hormone has been linked to increased risk of death in women with metastatic breast cancer.[95] Meditation can also help breast cancer patients and survivors fight off the depression and psychological stress that often go hand in hand with the disease.

In addition to reducing stress and developing a sense of inner peace, meditation can improve your memory and even increase your creativity. It's also been shown to fight inflammation and help with high blood pressure, heart disease, sleep problems, pain, addiction, and many other ailments.

Meditation is highly personal. Methods that work for others simply may not resonate with you. Search the web for different meditation practices until you find one you enjoy. You'll find many practitioners offer free guided meditations on their websites.

Start with a few minutes a day and work your way up to 20 minutes or more regularly. While you can definitely benefit from meditating for a few minutes, research has shown that 20 minutes a day can bring about the true magic.

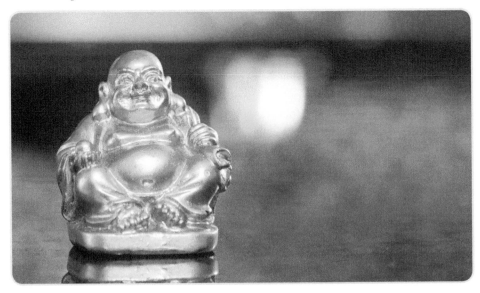

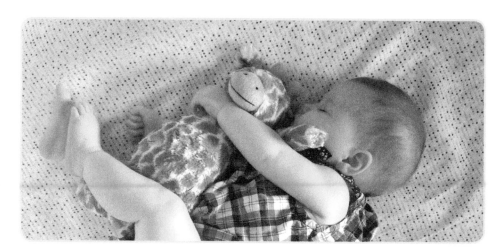

49 Savor Sleep

Ahhh, sleep—I love it! A good thing, because it's spectacularly good for human health.

Sleep has been linked to strengthening the immune system, losing weight, lowering stress levels, reducing feelings of depression, decreasing inflammation in our bodies and—you guessed it—lessening the chance of developing breast cancer.

Research supports this. An eight-year Japanese study that included 24,000 women showed those who regularly got six hours of sleep or less a night have a 62 percent greater chance of developing breast cancer than women who got seven hours a night.[96]

Another recent study found that getting six hours or less of sleep a night may increase the risk of breast cancer recurrence in post-menopausal women who've had the disease. In addition, the study also found a link between lack of sleep and having aggressive tumors.[97]

The connection between poor sleeping habits and breast cancer may also be related to the link between lack of sleep and obesity. It's well known that being obese puts you at a higher risk for breast cancer. Another reason may be insufficient levels of melatonin, a hormone that's produced by the brain while you sleep. Melatonin also suppresses the production of a particular type of estrogen linked to breast cancer.

If you're not yet convinced about the importance of sleep, keep in mind fatigue is believed to have been a major factor in both the Three Mile Island and Chernobyl nuclear disasters, with key operators allegedly falling asleep on the job.

How much sleep do you need? Experts say no magic number of hours works for everyone; it depends on your age, your health, and other factors. But as a general rule, seven to nine hours is the appropriate amount of sleep for an adult. If you currently sleep less than seven, increasing the time from that to nine hours all at once may be impossible. So start by increasing your sleep time in half-hour increments and let your body adjust until you reach a healthy number of hours.

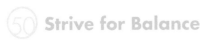# Strive for Balance

Sometimes, simply enjoying a pizza with friends is far more important than eating a kale salad alone. That's when you need to let go and have fun. Even if the meal isn't healthy, you're still nourishing your soul.

My goal in writing this book isn't to cause you stress and leave you feeling overwhelmed. As noted in the Introduction, you don't have to do all 50 of these tips every day. Instead, incorporate one tip a week over the course of the upcoming year. By taking incremental steps, you're far more likely to integrate important changes you can stay with for the long term.

Diving in headfirst and changing everything at once rarely works. Try each tip for one week. Then pick the ones that you want to stick and enjoy them!

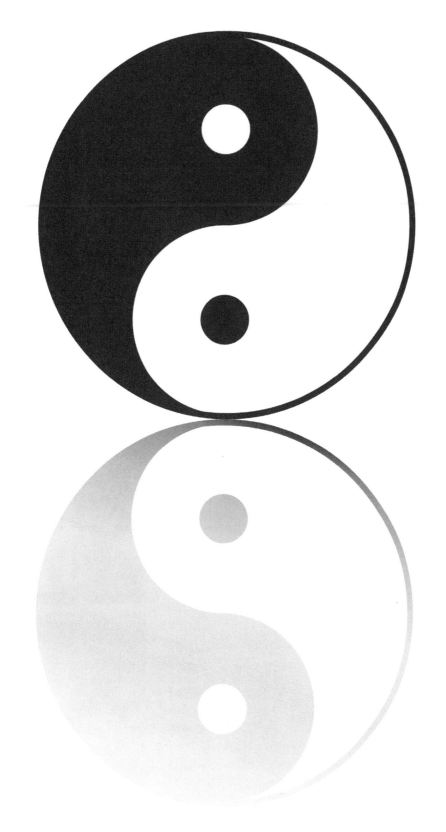

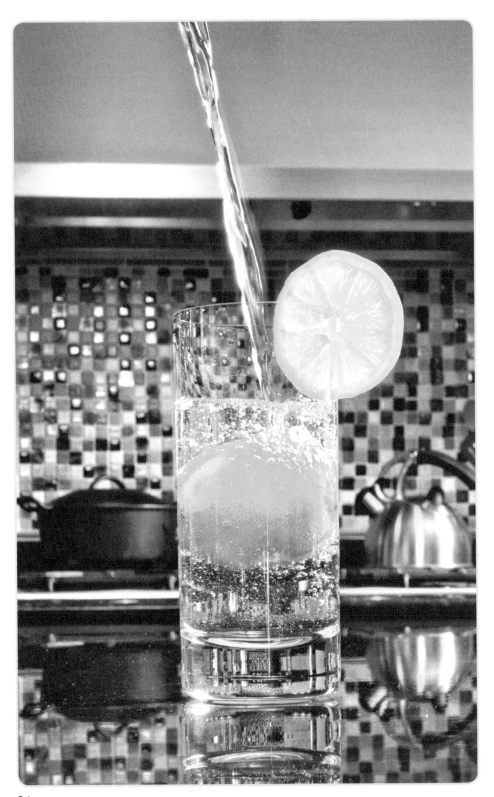

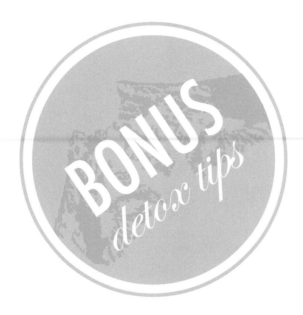

Full disclosure: Detoxing has lots of naysayers. Traditional doctors are often quick to point out that detoxing is unnecessary and potentially dangerous. They contend our bodies are designed to eliminate toxins automatically. In fact, our bodies are amazing machines that are highly skilled at booting out unwanted party guests.

However, it's quite possible they haven't adapted to—and simply cannot handle—the barrage of chemicals, GMOs, pesticides, radiation, and other nasties they're exposed to 24/7 in modern society.

Many holistic medical practitioners and some MDs believe that many of the diseases plaguing us (including cancer) are due in large part to toxicity in our bodies. They also believe we can assist our bodies in getting rid of built-up toxins.

Yes, your body is a perfectly designed detoxing machine, but with the abuse it gets these days, why not throw it a lifeline?

My advice is to strive to eat healthy, exercise often, drink lots of water, and pay attention to your environment. That means be careful of the things you put on your body, the air you breathe, and the water you drink. Treating your body like a garbage dump and then detoxing for several days may actually be dangerous. Many holistic health practitioners warn against rapid detox methods because the sudden onslaught of toxins into your bloodstream can make you very sick.

Therefore, I suggest that, on a regular basis, you engage in one or more of the following tips to give your body the detox break it may need.

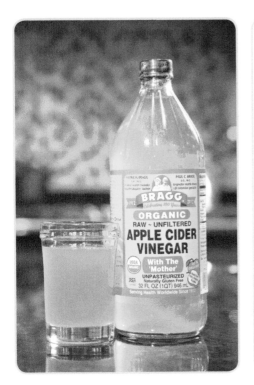
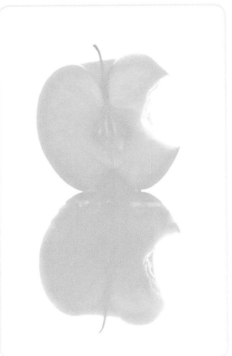

B①NUS tip **Admire ACV**

Apple cider vinegar is so versatile and has so many health benefits, it's hard to know where to start. Apple cider vinegar (ACV) is made from apples. The apples go through two stages of fermentation, first into hard cider and then into vinegar. One of its most potent health benefits is its ability to detoxify your body. Certain acids in ACV bind to toxins, thus allowing your body to flush them out. ACV also breaks up mucous in the body and cleanses the lymph nodes. This allows the lymph fluid to circulate properly and the lymph system overall to function as it should—removing toxins from the body and strengthening the immune system.

ACV also aids with acid reflux, boosts energy, gets rid of hiccups, fights yeast infections and other fungal conditions, controls blood sugar, lowers cholesterol, and aids digestion when taken before a meal.

To be honest, drinking apple cider vinegar is an acquired taste. It is vinegar, after all. Start by adding a teaspoon to a large glass of water and sipping it over several hours. Then work up to three teaspoons as you get accustomed to the taste.

As with most products, you'll find huge variations in quality. But even the best ACV is inexpensive, so go for the good stuff that's organic, unfiltered, and raw. Make sure it contains the "mother"—that weird looking chunk floating around in the bottle. (I consider the Bragg brand to be the king of ACV, available at grocery stores.)

B(2)NUS tip **Burn Your Bra**

This tip is a little whacky and not supported by scientific evidence. However, based on how constricting bras can feel, it makes a lot of sense. Some folks believe that tight-fitting bras may cut off lymph drainage, which could potentially lead to the development of breast cancer as well as benign cysts and lumps.

Plus, some evidence suggests that wearing a bra too often or too tight, or wearing an underwire bra, may be detrimental your health.

Back in 1995, the potential dangers of wearing a bra were highlighted in the book *Dressed to Kill: The Link Between Breast Cancer and Bras* by Sydney Ross Singer and Soma Grismaijer. The authors referenced a study of more than 4,000 women and concluded that women who do not wear bras have a much lower risk of breast cancer than those who do.

Specifically, the study found:

- ✿ Women who wore their bras 24 hours a day had a 3 out of 4 chance of developing breast cancer.

- ✿ Women who wore their bras more than 12 hours a day but not to bed had a 1 out of 7 risk of developing breast cancer.

- ✿ Women who wore their bras less than 12 hours a day had a 1 out of 52 risk of developing breast cancer.

- ✿ Women who wore bras rarely or never had a 1 out of 168 chance of getting breast cancer.

In addition, many Chinese medicine practitioners believe the metal in underwire bras interferes with your "chi" or healthy energy flow.

While you may not want to start an expensive bra-burning bonfire in a panic, consider taking the following steps to be cautious:

- ✿ Make sure your bra fits properly (this is just good advice, period).

- ✿ Minimize your time wearing underwire bras and consider replacing the metal wire with plastic. (You can find these for less than a dollar).

- ✿ Reduce the amount of time you spend in your bra altogether and, for gosh sakes, don't sleep in it!

And if you're worried about sagging breasts, a recent French study of women aged 18-35 showed that wearing a bra does not prevent sagging and may actually increase it.[98]

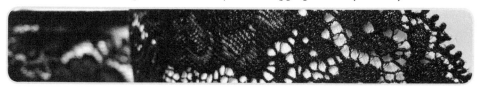

B③NUS tip **Delight in a Dip**

Taking a detox bath helps your body eliminate toxins and absorb any nutrients or minerals in the water. That's why one of the best additions to your bath is magnesium sulfate, also known as good old-fashioned Epsom salts.

Soaking in Epsom salts helps replenish your body's magnesium level. This is particularly important because approximately 70 percent of Americans are deficient in magnesium—one of the causes of high blood pressure. In addition, the sulfate flushes toxins from your body; plus Epsom salt baths help circulation and relax sore muscles and joints. Get in the bath after the salt has dissolved and be careful; the salt makes the bottom of the tub very slippery. Soak for at least 30 minutes; the longer you soak, the more minerals your body will absorb.

You could also add sodium bicarbonate or baking soda to your bath. Baking soda is anti-fungal, softens skin, and can neutralize the effects of radiation from x-rays, mammograms, and any of the other sources that bombard us daily. Soaking in a baking soda bath is also great after riding in an airplane—another source of radiation most people aren't aware of. Choose aluminum-free baking soda. Remember, aluminum is not your friend.

Adding apple cider vinegar is awesome in the tub. Not only does it draw toxins from your skin, it can improve your body's acid-alkaline balance. Add one to two cups of any or all of these ingredients listed.

Unmarked Obstacles

Safe Dipping

If you have heart problems, high blood pressure, diabetes, or other serious medical condition, consult your doctor before doing any of these baths. In addition, some people experience lightheadedness after bathing, so don't take these (or any other) baths when you're alone.

Besides, having company is also more fun.

For optimal bathing, use water that has been filtered to remove the chlorine at a medium-hot temperature. Water that's too hot strips the natural oils from your skin.

Relax, enjoy, and feel the stress melt away. For an extra special bath, add your favorite essential oils.

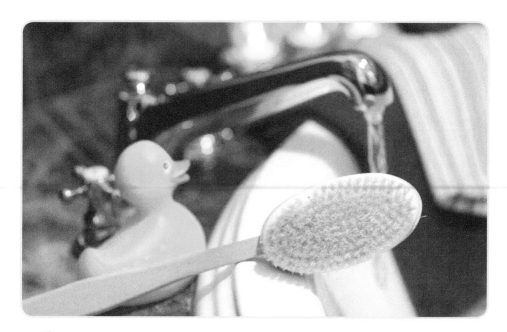

BONUS tip **Dig Your Dry Brush**

Did you know that your skin, as your body's largest organ, is responsible for one quarter of your natural detoxification each day? In fact, one to two pounds of waste is eliminated through your skin every single day. The skin is so crucial to your body's detoxification process, it's often referred to as the "second kidney."

To be clear, there are no studies specifically linking dry brushing to reduction in breast cancer. However, many in the natural health field believe the elimination of toxins from the body is crucial in preventing and treating disease, including breast cancer. This method has been used for centuries as a natural remedy in Scandinavia, Russia, and other parts of Europe, and is still common in European spas.

In addition to detoxification, you can enjoy the oodles of benefits that come with dry brushing. It:

- ❀ Increases circulation,

- ❀ Tones muscles,

- ❀ Helps digestion,

- ❀ Tones the skin and may reduce the appearance of cellulite,

- ❀ Eliminates dead skin cells and opens clogged pores,

- ❀ Improves nervous system functioning, and

- ❀ Stimulates internal organs through blood flow.

Want to give dry brushing a try? This process can take from one or two minutes up to 10 minutes. Follow these tips and your skin will be smooth and silky in no time:

- ❀ Make sure the brush and skin are dry.

- ❀ Use a brush with soft, natural bristles. No plastic or other synthetic brushes or loofas allowed!

- ❀ Start softly and increase pressure as your body gets accustomed to the process. Your skin should be pink or flushed when finished, not scratched, irritated, or in pain.

- ❀ Don't brush over any wounds, skin irritations, rashes, etc.

- ❀ Brush in straight motions going toward your heart. The only exceptions are your back and belly. Brush downward from your shoulders to your lower back and use a clockwise circular motion on your belly.

- ❀ Don't use a brush on your face; instead, use a dry washcloth.

- ❀ Avoid dry brushing your breasts.

- ❀ Clean the brush with soap and water often.

Take a shower after dry brushing, and if you can tolerate it, alternate hot and cold water in the shower to further increase blood circulation. After showering, towel dry and finish with a natural, chemical-free moisturizer or oil. (Coconut oil feels wonderful after dry brushing.)

This ritual will leave you feeling pampered and relaxed in no time!

Discovery Center

The Lymphatic System

While most folks know something about their circulatory system, very few know much about their lymphatic system. The two key jobs of the lymphatic system are:

- ❀ Distributing fluids, nutrients, and immune cells throughout the body, and

- ❀ Eliminating toxins and debris from your blood.

Your body has more lymph fluid than blood, but unlike the circulatory system, it doesn't come with a built-in pump (i.e., the ♥). Instead, the lymph system relies on skeletal muscle contractions or manual massage to move the fluid throughout your body. In addition to exercise, dry brushing accomplishes movement by stimulating the lymphatic system while it aids the skin in releasing toxins.

BONUS tip Love Lemon Water

Lemons are chock full of flavonoids, delivering top-notch benefits in the antioxidant, antibiotic, and anti-cancer departments. They are also antibacterial and antiviral. Lemons are loaded with vitamin C and help your body maintain proper pH levels; plus even a whiff of lemon can improve your concentration and brighten your mood.

As if that isn't enough, lemons also excel in the detox department. Starting each day with a glass of room-temperature water with the juice from half a lemon aids digestion, helps your body eliminate toxic waste, and even assists with constipation or diarrhea.

Interested in cutting your intake of caffeine? Think about how dehydrated you'd feel if you went seven to nine hours during the day without drinking water. That's the state we wake up in every morning. Unfortunately, many of us end up attempting to rehydrate with coffee or tea, which both have a dehydrating effect. Starting your day with a big glass of water is good practice, lemon or no lemon.

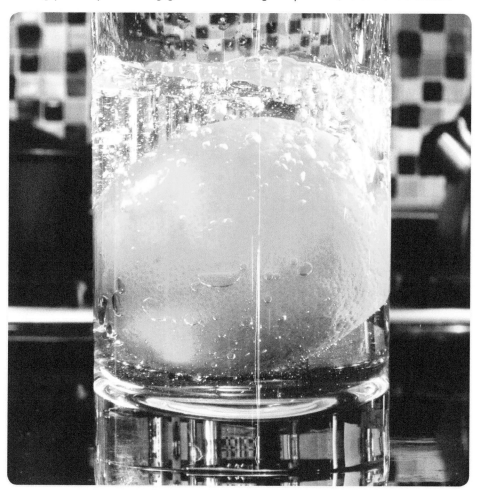

It has been my honor to share some of my favorite breast cancer prevention tips with you in this book. Thank you from the bottom of my heart.

Remember, small steps each day lead to major changes over the course of a few short months.

Start today.

– Kristina Sampson

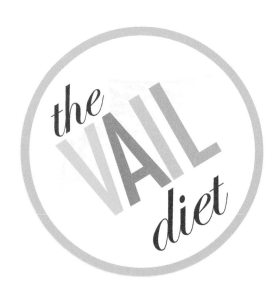

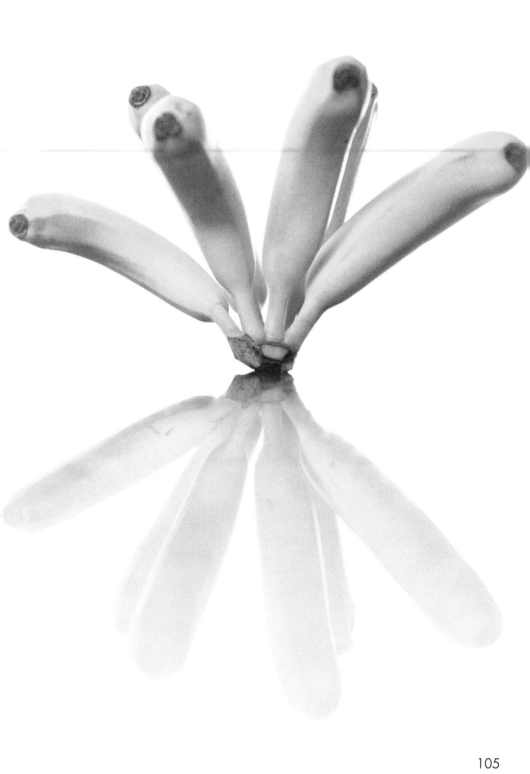

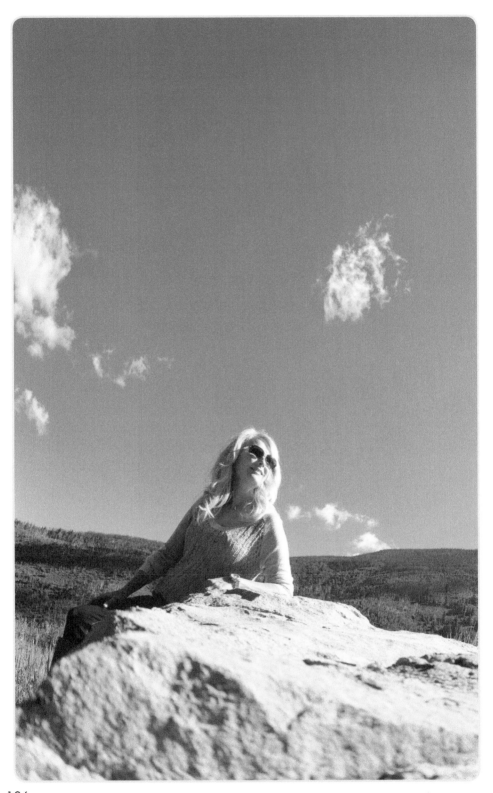

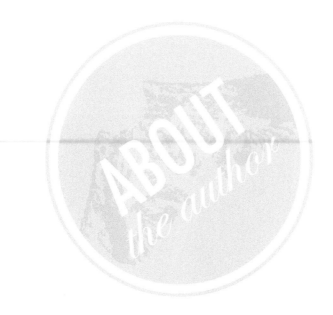

Kristina Sampson is a breast cancer survivor and CPA-turned-holistic health coach, certified by the Institute for Integrative Nutrition and the American Association of Drugless Practitioners. After her 2007 diagnosis of a rare and aggressive form of breast cancer, she took control of her well-being. While also undergoing traditional treatments, she brought her already healthy lifestyle to a whole new level. As a result of working with excellent doctors and living a "clean" lifestyle, Kristina has been happily cancer-free ever since.

This experience taught Kristina that life is too short to postpone following your passion. She decided to share The Vail Diet—the name she and her husband John coined to describe their treasured Colorado lifestyle—through her website and health coaching practice.

The Vail Diet focuses on eating real, nutrient-dense, high-quality food; reducing exposure to toxins in both your diet and your environment; being physically active; and incorporating your own unique approach to spirituality into your life.

Kristina's story appeared in the March 2014 issue of *Prevention Magazine*. She graduated from the Institute of Integrative Nutrition in July 2014 and will continue her nutrition education for the rest of her life.

To learn more about health coaching or invite Kristina to speak at your event, visit www.thevaildiet.com.

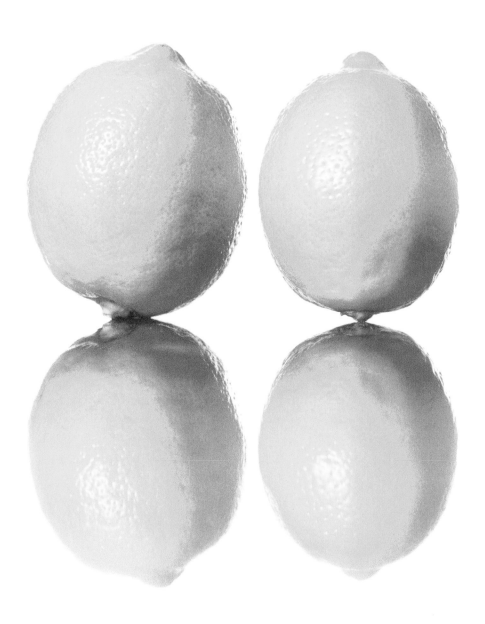

ACKNOWLEDGMENTS

While this book went from an idea to reality in only eight months, it encompasses a lifetime of influence and help from many important people in my life. At the top of this list is:

❋ My husband, John, whose support and encouragement gives me the space and freedom to pursue my dreams. If it weren't for him, Leave Cancer in the Dust may have never seen the light of day.

❋ My parents, Jim and Doris, for teaching me the importance of eating real food from an early age. They were way ahead of their time, discussing many of today's hottest nutrition topics since the 1970s. While I didn't always follow their advice in my younger days, when I was finally ready to settle down, I knew exactly where to land.

❋ My sister, Cherie, whose influence growing up turned me into a far more aware and interesting person than I may otherwise have been.

❋ My cousin, William (or Billy, as I know him) Sampson, whose artistic vision for the Vail Diet brought my ideas to life. His design and photography work on both my website and this book have brought them to a high level I couldn't have dreamed of.

❋ Siobhan O'Connor, Executive Editor of Prevention Magazine, for facilitating my appearance in Prevention. If it weren't for that event to light a spark under me, I might still be procrastinating starting this book. Prevention was part of our household for as long as I can remember; it was an honor to appear in the magazine.

❋ The Team of people who helped get Leave Cancer in the Dust out the door: Barbara McNichol (www.BarbaraMcNichol.com), whose great editing successfully removed the "noise" from my writing; Teresa Funke (www.TeresaFunke.com), who helped me clear several hurdles in one focused coaching session and was instrumental in creating the title; and Karen Saunders and Kelly Johnson (www.MacGraphics.net), who rescued me when I was paralyzed with uncertainty and indecision about the logistics of publishing.

Thank you all.

GLOSSARY
Learning Zone

Antioxidant – A substance that fights oxidative stress in the body, which can damage cellular DNA. DNA carries all of our genetic information.

Apoptosis – Fancy word for programmed cell "suicide." While that may sound scary, apoptosis is a natural process you *want* your cells to undergo. The damaged cells that cling to life wreak havoc on your body.

Carotenoids – Yellow, orange and red pigments in fruits and veggies that give them their beautiful colors. These include alpha-carotene, beta-carotene, and lutein, in addition to others. Carotenoids offer protection against breast cancer.

Ductal Carcinoma in Situ (DCIS) – Also known as "stage zero" breast cancer, DCIS is non-invasive breast cancer in which the abnormal cells are contained within the lining of the breast duct. If left untreated, DCIS can become an invasive form of the disease.

Endocrine system – Body system responsible for the production of hormones and critical for good health. Many of the endocrine system glands are located in the head and neck.

Estrogen – Female sex hormones produced mainly by the ovaries that are responsible for developing and maintaining female secondary sex characteristics. Secondary sex characteristics appear at puberty and differentiate between the sexes but aren't essential to reproduction (e.g., facial hair and breasts). Women produce three major types of estrogen—estrone, estradiol, and estriol.

Estrogen positive breast cancer (ER+) – Cancer consisting of cells with a significant number of estrogen receptors. The majority of breast cancers are ER+.

Flavanoids – Classes of plant pigments that act as antioxidants and scavenge DNA-damaging free radicals. They are found in fruits, veggies, nuts, seeds, and tea.

Flavanol – A class of flavonoids that occur naturally in a wide variety of fruits and veggies.

Free radical – In chemistry terms, this is an uncharged molecule with an unpaired valence electron. Because of the unpaired electron, free radicals are highly reactive and can damage DNA.

Glutathione peroxidase – Commonly called the body's "master antioxidant," this powerful substance protects the cells from oxidative stress and repairs damage to DNA.

Glycemic index – A system that ranks the carbohydrates in a food on a scale from 1 to 100. It's based on the average increase in blood sugar levels that occur after eating that carbohydrate. Foods with a high glycemic index may have a greater effect on blood sugar than those with a low glycemic index.

Glycemic load – While glycemic index measures the blood sugar effects of a carbohydrate in a particular food, glycemic load accounts for the amount of carbohydrate in that food. For instance, a carrot has a glycemic index of 35 but only has a glycemic load of 2, because a carrot is low in carbohydrates. Thus glycemic load is a more accurate indicator of glycemic response than the glycemic index because the glycemic index only measures the blood sugar *effect* of the carbs in a particular food. The *number* of carbs in that food is not a factor.

HER2/neu – An epidermal growth factor receptor that, when overexpressed, can cause a certain aggressive type of breast cancer.

Lymph – Lymph is a fluid in the body that circulates and collects unwanted materials, which are then filtered through the lymphatic system. Our bodies have more than three times more lymph than blood, yet unlike blood, lymph does not come with its own pump. Rather, it depends on movement within the body for proper flow.

Meta-analysis – A study that reviews and compiles the results of many different studies.

Oleic acid – Monounsaturated fat found in a variety of both plant and animal fats and oils. Women who include a lot of this healthy monounsaturated fat in their diet have been shown to have lower rates of breast cancer. Olive oil is a good source of this important acid.

Oxidation – The chemical reaction that occurs when a substance combines with oxygen. Oxidation causes apples, pears, bananas, avocados, and other fruits to turn brown when exposed to air and also causes metal to rust. It damages our DNA.

Phytochemicals – Biologically active compounds found in plants. Flavonoids, carotenoids, and lignans are only a few of the thousands of phytochemicals that have been identified in plants.

Phytoestrogens – A naturally occurring compound in certain plants that acts as an estrogen in the body. Hundreds of plants contain phytoestrogens including soybeans, legumes, flaxseeds, beans, cereal brans, sesame seeds, sunflower seeds, pistachio nuts, walnuts, winter squash, broccoli, cabbage, peaches, apples, and strawberries.

Progesterone – Female sex hormone that regulates the menstrual cycle and supports pregnancy.

T-Cells – These cells play a crucial role in our immune response and are major cancer fighters.

Triple negative breast cancer – Cancer consisting of cells that are estrogen and progesterone receptor negative, as well as HER2/neu negative. Approximately 10 to 20 percent of breast cancers are triple negative. This type of breast cancer is considered by doctors as being hard to treat because it does not respond to common therapies such as Tamoxifen and Herceptin.

ENDNOTES

1- American Cancer Society. Cancer Facts & Figures 2013-2014. Atlanta: American Cancer Society; 2013.

2- Anand P, et al. Cancer is a preventable disease that requires major lifestyle changes. Pharm Res. 2008 Sep;25(9):2097-116. doi: 10.1007/s11095-008-9661-9. Epub 2008 Jul 15. Review. Erratum in: Pharm Res. 2008 Sep;25(9):2200. Kunnumakara, Ajaikumar B. PubMed PMID: 18626751; PubMed Central PMCID: PMC2515569.

3- Crystal Smith-Spangler, et al. Are Organic Foods Safer or Healthier Than Conventional Alternatives? A Systematic Review. Annals of Internal Medicine. 2012 Sep;157(5):348-366.

4- Brandt K, et al. "Agroecosystem management and nutritional quality of plant foods: The case of organic fruits and vegetables." Newcastle University. http://www.ncl.ac.uk/afrd/research/publication/168871 (accessed January 2, 2014).

5- Food for Breast Cancer. "Studies Have Not Established the Effect of Beets on Breast Cancer." Food for Breast Cancer. http://foodforbreastcancer.com/foods/beets (accessed December 31, 2013).

6- Reddy MK, et al. Relative inhibition of lipid peroxidation, cyclooxygenase enzymes, and human tumor cell proliferation by natural food colors. J Agric Food Chem. 2005 Nov 16;53(23):9268-73. PubMed PMID: 16277432.

7- Mafuvadze B, et al. Apigenin induces apoptosis and blocks growth of medroxyprogesterone acetate-dependent BT-474 xenograft tumors. Horm Cancer. 2012 Aug;3(4):160-71. doi: 10.1007/s12672-012-0114-x. Epub 2012 May 9. PubMed PMID: 22569706.

8- Timothy Wall. "Breast Cancer Effectively Treated With Chemical Found in Celery, Parsley by MU Researchers." University of Missouri. http://munews.missouri.edu/news-releases/2012/0515-breast-cancer-effectively-treated-with-chemical-found-in-celery-parsley-and-spice-by-mu-researchers/ (accessed December 31, 2013).

9- Li Y, Zhang T. Targeting cancer stem cells with sulforaphane, a dietary component from broccoli and broccoli sprouts. Future Oncol. 2013 Aug;9(8):1097-103. doi: 10.2217/fon.13.108. PubMed PMID: 23902242.

10-Author unknown. "Eating Cruciferous Vegetables May Improve Breast Cancer Survival." Vanderbilt University Medical Center. http://www.mc.vanderbilt.edu/news/releases.php?release=2395 (accessed January 11, 2014).

11-Syed Alwi SS, et al. In vivo modulation of 4E binding protein 1 (4E-BP1) phosphorylation by watercress: a pilot study. Br J Nutr. 2010 Nov;104(9):1288-96. doi: 10.1017/S0007114510002217. Epub 2010 Jun 15. PubMed PMID: 20546646; PubMed Central PMCID: PMC3694331.

12-Galeone C, et al. Onion and garlic use and human cancer. Am J Clin Nutr. 2006 Nov;84(5):1027-32. PubMed PMID: 17093154. http://ajcn.nutrition. org/content/84/5/1027.long

13-Challier B, et al. Garlic, onion and cereal fibre as protective factors for breast cancer: a French case-control study. Eur J Epidemiol. 1998 Dec;14(8):737-47. PubMed PMID: 9928867.

14-Joy Bauer. "10 Best Foods for Cancer Prevention." JoyBauer.com. http:// www.joybauer.com/photo-gallery/10-best-foods-for-cancer-prevention/Sweet-potatoes.aspx (accessed December 31, 2013).

15-Zhang X, et al. Carotenoid intakes and risk of breast cancer defined by estrogen receptor and progesterone receptor status: a pooled analysis of 18 prospective cohort studies. Am J Clin Nutr. 2012 Mar;95(3):713-25. doi: 10.3945/ajcn.111.014415. Epub 2012 Jan 25. PubMed PMID: 22277553; PubMed Central PMCID: PMC3278246.

16-Nutrition Action Health Letter. "10 Worst and Best Foods." Centers for Science in the Public Interest. http://www.cspinet.org/nah/10foods_bad.html (accessed January 8, 2014).

17-Mark Hyman. "What is Glutathione and How Do I Get More of It?" drhyman.com. http://drhyman.com/blog/2010/05/12/what-is-glutathione-and-how-do-i-get-more-of-it/ (accessed December 31, 2013).

18-Blanche Levine. "The Health Benefits of Avocado Prevent and Reverse Cancer." NaturalHealth365.com. http://www.naturalhealth365.com/food_news/reverse_cancer.html (accessed December 31, 2013).

19-Boyer J, Liu RH. Apple phytochemicals and their health benefits. Nutr J. 2004 May 12;3:5. PubMed PMID: 15140261; PubMed Central PMCID: PMC442131.

20-Author unknown. "Apples Could Help Reduce the Risk of Breast Cancer." Cornell University College of Agriculture and Life Sciences. http://impact. cals.cornell.edu/project/apples-could-help-reduce-risk-breast-cancer (accessed December 31, 2013).

21-Fung TT, et al. Intake of specific fruits and vegetables in relation to risk of estrogen receptor-negative breast cancer among postmenopausal women. Breast Cancer Res Treat. 2013 Apr;138(3):925-30. doi: 10.1007/s10549-013-2484-3. Epub 2013 Mar 27. PubMed PMID: 23532538; PubMed Central PMCID: PMC3641647.

22-Adams LS, et al. Blueberry phytochemicals inhibit growth and metastatic potential of MDA-MB-231 breast cancer cells through modulation of the phosphatidylinositol 3-kinase pathway. Cancer Res. 2010 May 1;70(9):3594-605. doi: 10.1158/0008-5472.CAN-09-3565. Epub 2010 Apr 13. PubMed PMID: 20388778; PubMed Central PMCID: PMC2862148.

23-Noratto G, et al. Identifying peach and plum polyphenols with chemopreventive potential against estrogen-independent breast cancer cells. J Agric Food Chem. 2009 Jun 24;57(12):5219-26. doi: 10.1021/jf900259m. PubMed PMID: 19530711.

24-Rossato SB, et al. Antioxidant potential of peels and fleshes of peaches from different cultivars. J Med Food. 2009 Oct;12(5):1119-26. doi: 10.1089/jmf.2008.0267. PubMed PMID: 19857078.

25-Adams LS, et al. Pomegranate ellagitannin-derived compounds exhibit antiproliferative and antiaromatase activity in breast cancer cells in vitro. Cancer Prev Res (Phila). 2010 Jan;3(1):108-13. doi: 10.1158/1940-6207. CAPR-08-0225. PubMed PMID: 20051378; PubMed Central PMCID: PMC2805471.

26-Rocha A, et al. Pomegranate juice and specific components inhibit cell and molecular processes critical for metastasis of breast cancer. Breast Cancer Res Treat. 2012 Dec;136(3):647-58. doi: 10.1007/s10549-012-2264-5. Epub 2012 Oct 12. PubMed PMID: 23065001.

27-Jeune MA, et al. Anticancer activities of pomegranate extracts and genistein in human breast cancer cells. J Med Food. 2005 Winter;8(4):469-75. PubMed PMID: 16379557.

28-Lee HS, et al. [6]-Gingerol inhibits metastasis of MDA-MB-231 human breast cancer cells. J Nutr Biochem. 2008 May;19(5):313-9. Epub 2007 Aug 1. PubMed PMID: 17683926.

29-Elkady AI, et al. Differential control of growth, apoptotic activity, and gene expression in human breast cancer cells by extracts derived from medicinal herbs Zingiber officinale. J Biomed Biotechnol. 2012;2012:614356. doi: 10.1155/2012/614356. Epub 2012 Aug 26. PubMed PMID: 22969274; PubMed Central PMCID: PMC3433172.

30-Yekta ZP, et al. Ginger as a miracle against chemotherapy-induced vomiting. Iran J Nurs Midwifery Res. 2012 Jul;17(5):325-9. PubMed PMID: 23853643; PubMed Central PMCID: PMC3703071.

31-Johnson JJ. Carnosol: a promising anti-cancer and anti-inflammatory agent. Cancer Lett. 2011 Jun 1;305(1):1-7. doi: 10.1016/j.canlet.2011.02.005. Epub 2011 Mar 5. Review. PubMed PMID: 21382660; PubMed Central PMCID: PMC3070765.

32-Ngo SN, et al. Rosemary and cancer prevention: preclinical perspectives. Crit Rev Food Sci Nutr. 2011 Dec;51(10):946-54. doi: 10.1080/10408398.2010.490883. Review. PubMed PMID: 21955093.

33-Zhu BT, et al. Dietary administration of an extract from rosemary leaves enhances the liver microsomal metabolism of endogenous estrogens and decreases their uterotropic action in CD-1 mice. Carcinogenesis. 1998 Oct;19(10):1821-7. PubMed PMID: 9806165.

34-Chryssanthi DG, et al. Crocetin inhibits invasiveness of MDA-MB-231 breast cancer cells via downregulation of matrix metalloproteinases. Planta Med. 2011 Jan;77(2):146-51. doi: 10.1055/s-0030-1250178. Epub 2010 Aug 27. PubMed PMID: 20803418.

35-Aggarwal S, et al. Curcumin (diferuloylmethane) down-regulates expression of cell proliferation and antiapoptotic and metastatic gene products through suppression of IkappaBalpha kinase and Akt activation. Mol Pharmacol. 2006 Jan;69(1):195-206. Epub 2005 Oct 11. PubMed PMID: 16219905.

36-Kakarala M, et al. Targeting breast stem cells with the cancer preventive compounds curcumin and piperine. Breast Cancer Res Treat. 2010 Aug;122(3):777-85. doi: 10.1007/s10549-009-0612-x. Epub 2009 Nov 7. PubMed PMID: 19898931; PubMed Central PMCID: PMC3039120.

37-http://www.mce.k12tn.net/chocolate/history/history_of_chocolate1.htm (accessed January 8, 2014).

38-Ramljak D, et al. Pentameric procyanidin from Theobroma cacao selectively inhibits growth of human breast cancer cells. Mol Cancer Ther. 2005 Apr;4(4):537-46. PubMed PMID: 15827326.

39-Author unknown. "Lignans." Linus Pauling Institute. http://lpi.oregonstate.edu/infocenter/phytochemicals/lignans/ (accessed January 8, 2014).

40-Flower G, et al. Flax and Breast Cancer: A Systematic Review. Integr Cancer Ther. 2013 Sep 8. [Epub ahead of print] PubMed PMID: 24013641.

41-Adebamowo CA, et al. Dietary flavonols and flavonol-rich foods intake and the risk of breast cancer. Int J Cancer. 2005 Apr 20;114(4):628-33. PubMed PMID: 15609322.

42-Thompson MD, et al. Mechanisms associated with dose-dependent inhibition of rat mammary carcinogenesis by dry bean (Phaseolus vulgaris, L.). J Nutr. 2008 Nov;138(11):2091-7. doi: 10.3945/jn.108.094557. PubMed PMID: 18936203.

43-McCullough, Marji. "The Bottom Line on Soy and Breast Cancer Risk." American Cancer Society. http://www.cancer.org/cancer/news/expertvoices/post/2012/08/02/the-bottom-line-on-soy-and-breast-cancer-risk.aspx (accessed January 14, 2014).

44-Kang X, et al. Effect of soy isoflavones on breast cancer recurrence and death for patients receiving adjuvant endocrine therapy. CMAJ. 2010 Nov 23;182(17):1857-62. doi: 10.1503/cmaj.091298. Epub 2010 Oct 18. PubMed PMID: 20956506; PubMed Central PMCID: PMC2988534.

45-Berkey CS, et al. Vegetable protein and vegetable fat intakes in pre-adolescent and adolescent girls, and risk for benign breast disease in young women. Breast Cancer Res Treat. 2013 Sep;141(2):299-306. doi: 10.1007/s10549-013-2686-8. Epub 2013 Sep 17. PubMed PMID: 24043428.

46-Hardman WE, et al. Dietary walnut suppressed mammary gland tumorigenesis in the C(3)1 TAg mouse. Nutr Cancer. 2011;63(6):960-70. doi: 10.1080/01635581.2011.589959. Epub 2011 Jul 20. PubMed PMID: 21774594; PubMed Central PMCID: PMC3474134.

47-Ingram D, et al. Case-control study of phyto-oestrogens and breast cancer. Lancet. 1997 Oct 4;350(9083):990-4. PubMed PMID: 9329514.

48-Garland CF, et al. Vitamin D and prevention of breast cancer: pooled analysis. J Steroid Biochem Mol Biol. 2007 Mar;103(3-5):708-11. PubMed PMID: 17368188.

49-Garland CF, et al. Vitamin D for cancer prevention: global perspective. Ann Epidemiol. 2009 Jul;19(7):468-83. doi: 10.1016/j.annepidem.2009.03.021. Review. PubMed PMID: 19523595.

50-Mercola, Joseph. "The Wonder Vitamin That May Help You Prevent 16 Types of Cancer." Mercola.com. http://articles.mercola.com/sites/articles/archive/2011/10/22/carole-baggerly-on-vitamin-d.aspx (accessed January 15, 2014).

51-Yamamoto S, et al; Japan Public Health Center-Based Prospective Study on Cancer Cardiovascular Diseases Group. Soy, isoflavones, and breast cancer risk in Japan. J Natl Cancer Inst. 2003 Jun 18;95(12):906-13. PubMed PMID: 12813174.

52-Author unknown. "Tea and Cancer Prevention: Strengths and Limits of the Evidence." National Cancer Institute. http://www.cancer.gov/cancertopics/factsheet/prevention/tea (accessed January 1, 2014).

53-Sun CL, et al. Green tea, black tea and breast cancer risk: a meta-analysis of epidemiological studies. Carcinogenesis. 2006 Jul;27(7):1310-5. Epub 2005 Nov 25. PubMed PMID: 16311246.

54-Zheng JS, et al. Intake of fish and marine n-3 polyunsaturated fatty acids and risk of breast cancer: meta-analysis of data from 21 independent prospective cohort studies. BMJ. 2013 Jun 27;346:f3706. doi: 10.1136/bmj.f3706. Review. PubMed PMID: 23814120.

55-Xiong A, et al. Distinct roles of different forms of vitamin E in DHA-induced apoptosis in triple-negative breast cancer cells. Mol Nutr Food Res. 2012 Jun;56(6):923-34. doi: 10.1002/mnfr.201200027. PubMed PMID: 22707267.

56-Altenburg JD, Siddiqui RA. Omega-3 polyunsaturated fatty acids down-modulate CXCR4 expression and function in MDA-MB-231 breast cancer cells. Mol Cancer Res. 2009 Jul;7(7):1013-20. doi: 10.1158/1541-7786.MCR-08-0385. Epub 2009 Jun 30. PubMed PMID: 19567784.

57-Zhang M, Huang J, Xie X, Holman CD. Dietary intakes of mushrooms and green tea combine to reduce the risk of breast cancer in Chinese women. Int J Cancer. 2009 Mar 15;124(6):1404-8. doi: 10.1002/ijc.24047. PubMed PMID: 19048616.

58-Hamajima N, et al. for the Collaborative Group on Hormonal Factors in Breast Cancer. Alcohol, tobacco and breast cancer–collaborative reanalysis of individual data from 53 epidemiological studies, including 58,515 women with breast cancer and 95,067 women without the disease. Br J Cancer. 2002 Nov 18;87(11):1234-45. PubMed PMID: 12439712; PubMed Central PMCID: PMC2562507.

59-Liu Y, et al. Alcohol intake between menarche and first pregnancy: a prospective study of breast cancer risk. J Natl Cancer Inst. 2013 Oct 16;105(20):1571-8. doi: 10.1093/jnci/djt213. Epub 2013 Aug 28. PubMed PMID: 23985142; PubMed Central PMCID: PMC3797023.

60-Kohlmeier L, et al. Adipose tissue trans fatty acids and breast cancer in the European Community Multicenter Study on Antioxidants, Myocardial Infarction, and Breast Cancer. Cancer Epidemiol Biomarkers Prev. 1997 Sep;6(9):705-10. PubMed PMID: 9298578.

61-Chajès V, et al. Association between serum trans-monounsaturated fatty acids and breast cancer risk in the E3N-EPIC Study. Am J Epidemiol. 2008 Jun 1;167(11):1312-20. doi: 10.1093/aje/kwn069. Epub 2008 Apr 4. PubMed PMID: 18390841; PubMed Central PMCID: PMC2679982.

62-Gaudet MM, et al. Active smoking and breast cancer risk: original cohort data and meta-analysis. J Natl Cancer Inst. 2013 Apr 17;105(8):515-25. doi: 10.1093/jnci/djt023. Epub 2013 Feb 28. PubMed PMID: 23449445.

63-Minger, Denise. "The China Study: Fact or Fallacy?" Raw Food SOS. http://rawfoodsos.com/2010/07/07/the-china-study-fact-or-fallac/ (accessed January 2, 2014).

64-Author unknown. "Lactose Intolerance." U.S. National Library of Medicine. http://ghr.nlm.nih.gov/condition/lactose-intolerance (accessed January 8, 2014).

65-Kim YI. Does a high folate intake increase the risk of breast cancer? Nutr Rev. 2006 Oct;64(10 Pt 1):468-75. Review. PubMed PMID: 17063929.

66-Figueiredo JC, et al. Folic acid and risk of prostate cancer: results from a randomized clinical trial. J Natl Cancer Inst. 2009 Mar 18;101(6):432-5. doi: 10.1093/jnci/djp019. Epub 2009 Mar 10. PubMed PMID: 19276452; PubMed Central PMCID: PMC2657096.

67-Kaaks R, et al. Insulin-like growth factor I and risk of breast cancer by age and hormone receptor status-A prospective study within the EPIC cohort. Int J Cancer. 2013 Nov 7. doi: 10.1002/ijc.28589. [Epub ahead of print] PubMed PMID: 24248481.

68-Author unknown. "Red and Processed Meats and Cancer Prevention." World Cancer Research Fund. http://www.wcrf-uk.org/cancer_prevention/recommendations/meat_and_cancer.php (accessed January 8, 2014).

69-Rohrmann S, et al. Meat consumption and mortality–results from the European Prospective Investigation into Cancer and Nutrition. BMC Med. 2013 Mar 7;11:63. doi: 10.1186/1741-7015-11-63. PubMed PMID: 23497300; PubMed Central PMCID: PMC3599112.

70-Author unknown. "GMO Facts." Non-GMO Project. http://www.nongmoproject.org/learn-more/ (accessed January 8, 2014).

71-Vrain, T. (2013, June 7). The Gene Revolution, The Future of Agriculture: Dr. Thierry Vrain at TEDxComoxValley. Retrieved from http://www.youtube.com/watch?v=RQkQXyiynYs.

72-Séralini GE, et al. Long term toxicity of a Roundup herbicide and a Roundup-tolerant genetically modified maize. Food Chem Toxicol. 2012 Nov;50(11):4221-31. doi: 10.1016/j.fct.2012.08.005. Epub 2012 Sep 19. PubMed PMID: 22999595.

73-Pollan, Michael. "Playing God in the Garden," New York Times Magazine, October 25, 1998.

74-Ayala, Cesar J. American Sugar Kingdom: The Plantation Economy of the Spanish Caribbean, 1898-1934. The University of North Carolina Press, 1999.

75-Arcidiacono B, et al. Insulin resistance and cancer risk: an overview of the pathogenetic mechanisms. Exp Diabetes Res. 2012;2012:789174. doi: 10.1155/2012/789174. Epub 2012 Jun 4. Review. PubMed PMID: 22701472; PubMed Central PMCID: PMC3372318.

76-Favero A, et al. Energy sources and risk of cancer of the breast and colon-rectum in Italy. Adv Exp Med Biol. 1999;472:51-5. PubMed PMID: 10736615.

77-Reynolds, Gretchen. "Don't Just Sit There," *The New York Times*, April 28, 2012, online edition.

78-Morris JN, et al. Coronary heart-disease and physical activity of work. Lancet. 1953 Nov 28;265(6796):1111-20; concl. PubMed PMID: 13110075.

79-Hellmich, Nanci. "Prolonged Sitting Linked to Breast Cancer, Colon Cancer," *USA Today*, November 3, 2011, online edition.

80-Wilmot EG, et al. Sedentary time in adults and the association with diabetes, cardiovascular disease and death: systematic review and meta-analysis. Diabetologia. 2012 Nov;55(11):2895-905. doi: 10.1007/s00125-012-2677-z. Epub 2012 Aug 14. Review. Erratum in: Diabetologia. 2013 Apr;56(4):942-3. PubMed PMID: 22890825.

81-Ahmed RL, et al. Randomized controlled trial of weight training and lymphedema in breast cancer survivors. J Clin Oncol. 2006 Jun 20;24(18):2765-72. Epub 2006 May 15. Erratum in: J Clin Oncol. 2006 Aug 1;24(22):3716. PubMed PMID: 16702582.

82-Simon, Stacy. "Study Links Walking to Lower Breast Cancer Risk." American Cancer Society. http://www.cancer.org/cancer/news/study-links-walking-to-lower-breast-cancer-risk (accessed January 1, 2014).

83-Jain R, et al. Clinical Studies Examining the Impact of Obesity on Breast Cancer Risk and Prognosis. J Mammary Gland Biol Neoplasia. 2013 Nov 13. [Epub ahead of print] PubMed PMID: 24221746.

84-Author unknown. "BMI Calculator." Prevention.com. http://www.prevention.com/fitness/fitness-tips/bmi-calculator (accessed January 1, 2014).

85-Sifferlin, Alexandra. "Dropping a Few Pounds Could Lower Breast Cancer Risk." *Time Magazine*, (May 22, 2012), http://healthland.time.com/2012/05/22/dropping-a-few-pounds-could-lower-breast-cancer-risk/.

86-Levine AS, Balk JL. Pilot study of yoga for breast cancer survivors with poor quality of life. Complement Ther Clin Pract. 2012 Nov;18(4):241-5. doi: 10.1016/j.ctcp.2012.06.007. Epub 2012 Aug 3. PubMed PMID: 23059439.

87-Author unknown. "Antiperspirants/Deodorants and Breast Cancer." National Cancer Institute. http://www.cancer.gov/cancertopics/factsheet/Risk/AP-Deo (accessed January 1, 2014).

88-Author unknown. "National Drinking Water Database." Environmental Working Group. http://www.ewg.org/tap-water/ (accessed January 1, 2014).

89-Author unknown. "Study Reports on Cleaning Products, Beliefs About Breast Cancer, and Breast Cancer Risk." Silent Spring Institute. http://www.silentspring.org/our-research/research-updates/study-reports-cleaning-products-beliefs-about-breast-cancer-and-breast (accessed January 1, 2014).

90-Walsh, Bryan. "Why the FDA Hasn't Banned Potentially Toxic BPA (Yet)." *Time Magazine*, (April 3, 2012), http://content.time.com/time/health/article/0,8599,2110902,00.html.

91-Stokes, Paul. "Body Absorbs 5lb of Makeup Chemicals a Year." *The Telegraph*, June 21, 2007, online edition. http://www.telegraph.co.uk/news/uknews/1555173/Body-absorbs-5lb-of-make-up-chemicals-a-year.html

92-Barr L, et al. Measurement of paraben concentrations in human breast tissue at serial locations across the breast from axilla to sternum. J Appl Toxicol. 2012 Mar;32(3):219-32. doi: 10.1002/jat.1786. Epub 2012 Jan 12. PubMed PMID: 22237600.

93-Hernandez-Reif M, et al. Breast cancer patients have improved immune and neuroendocrine functions following massage therapy. J Psychosom Res. 2004 Jul;57(1):45-52. PubMed PMID: 15256294.

94-Yang, Sarah. "To Revert Breast Cancer Cells, Give Them a Squeeze." UC Berkeley News Center. http://newscenter.berkeley.edu/2012/12/17/malignant-breast-cells-grow-normally-when-compressed/(accessed January 1, 2014).

95-Sephton SE, et al. Diurnal cortisol rhythm as a predictor of breast cancer survival. J Natl Cancer Inst. 2000 Jun 21;92(12):994-1000. PubMed PMID: 10861311.

96-Irvine, Chris. "Less Than Six Hours Sleep a Night Raises Breast Cancer Risk by 60 Percent." *The Telegraph*, November 3, 2008, online edition. http://www.telegraph.co.uk/health/3369361/Less-than-six-hours-sleep-a-night-raises-breast-cancer-risk-by-60-per-cent.html

97-Author unknown. "Lack of Sleep Found to be a New Risk Factor for Aggressive Breast Cancers." University Hospitals. http://www.uhhospitals.org/about/media-news-room/current-news/2012/08/lack-of-sleep-found-to-be-a-new-risk-factor-for-aggressive-breast-cancers (accessed January 1, 2014).

98-Castillo, Michelle. "French Study Suggests Younger Women Should Stop Wearing Bras." CBS News. http://www.cbsnews.com/news/french-study-suggests-younger-women-should-stop-wearing-bras/ (accessed January 1, 2014).

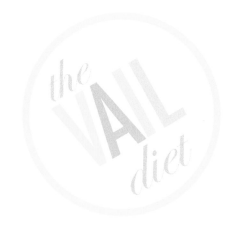

Want more?

If you enjoyed this book, please join my e-mail list
to receive more mind nourishing content.

www.thevaildiet.com

Or follow me on your favorite form of social media:

facebook.com

twitter.com

pinterest.com   /thevaildiet

instagram.com

youtube.com

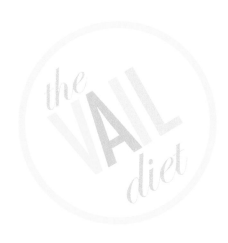